KIDNEY FAILURE EXPLAINED

Everything you always wanted to know
about dialysis and kidney transplants
but were afraid to ask

Sixth Edition

KIDNEY FAILURE EXPLAINED

Everything you always wanted to know
about dialysis and kidney transplants
but were afraid to ask

Sixth Edition

Janet Wild, *RGN, PG CertMedEd*
Market Access and Therapy Development Manager, Baxter Healthcare Ltd, Newbury, Berkshire

Dr Richard Fluck, *FRCP, MA (Cantab), MBBS*
Consultant Renal Physician, Royal Derby Hospital

CLASS HEALTH • BRIDGWATER

Printing history
This edition – Authors: Janet Wild and Richard Fluck
First published 2019
Reprinted 2019

Previous editions:
First published 1999 – Authors: Andy Stein and Janet Wild
Second edition 2002 – Authors: Andy Stein and Janet Wild
Third edition 2007 – Authors: Andy Stein and Janet Wild
Fourth edition 2010 – Authors: Andy Stein and Janet Wild
Fifth edition 2017 – Authors: Janet Wild and Richard Fluck

The authors and publisher welcome feedback from the users of this book. Please contact the publisher:

Class Health, The Exchange, Express Park, Bridgwater, Somerset TA6 4RR
Tel: 44(0)1278 427800
Email: post@class.co.uk
Website: www.classhealth.co.uk

The information presented in this book is accurate and current to the best of the authors' knowledge. The authors and publisher, however, make no guarantee as to, and assume no responsibility for, the correctness, sufficiency or completeness of such information or recommendation. The reader is advised to consult a doctor regarding all aspects of individual health care.

Class Health is an imprint of Class Publishing Ltd.

A CIP catalogue for this book is available from the British Library.

ISBN 978-1-85959-792-7
Ebook ISBN 978-1-85959-793-4

10 9 8 7 6 5 4 3 2 1

Edited by Shanon Rademacher
Illustrations by Darren Bennett and David Woodroffe
Typeset by RefineCatch Limited, Bungay, Suffolk
Printed in Great Britain by Ashford Colour Press

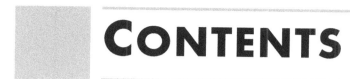

CONTENTS

FOREWORD

Having read this latest 2019 version of *Kidney Failure Explained*, I realise just how much things have moved on in our world of kidney disease in the last few years.

As a kidney patient of some 30 years now I know that knowledge is confidence. It is the difference between just accepting what is being said to you and getting on with it, and having the confidence to engage and sometimes challenge decisions about your treatment care and ultimately your chances of enjoying a long life. We are individuals, each with a very different take on what the words 'acceptable quality of life' mean.

I remember being asked if I had any questions just moments after finding out that my native kidneys were failing back in 1989 after a long spell of feeling so weak and ill, and just not knowing what to ask – because I knew nothing. I might have come back with a list of questions had I had access to this publication back then, and certainly would not have made some of the choices I made then when considering my treatment options.

This edition of *Kidney Failure Explained* explains what is happening to our body as our kidneys fail, the daily issues we face and those long-term decisions which affect not just us but those around us who love and care for us, head on. It is written in a no-nonsense, intelligent way that just says it as it is. Chronic Kidney Disease (CKD) is forever ('chronic') and often a frightening and isolating experience. Whether you're dialysing or have a successful transplant, you are, like it or not, a kidney patient for life. For me, the only way to deal with this reality is to learn as much as I possibly can about my condition, its treatment, how to access and accept help if I need it and what I can do to enhance my chances of living a long and reasonably healthy life. I found that information in *Kidney Failure Explained*.

As an Editor of Kidney Matters (a Kidney Care UK quarterly publication) and Lead on the Kidney Kitchen project, I have also found this publication immensely helpful and informative. If you are not up to reading whole chapters then I recommend you read at least the Key Facts at the end of each chapter. You WILL need the information listed there as you take-on CKD and all the challenges – and triumphs it can bring.

Kidney Failure Explained is now my 'go to' reference book and I thank Janet Wild and Richard Fluck for putting in the hours to get it published.

Deborah Duval
Managing Editor
Kidney Care UK

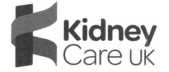

FOREWORD

There is so much misunderstanding about kidney disease, even amongst those who have been diagnosed with it. This is a real concern as latest figures indicate that there are 3 million people in the UK with chronic kidney disease. So *Kidney Failure Explained*, with its comprehensive explanations and clear diagrams, is greatly needed.

Chronic kidney disease is complex and therefore treatments and preventative measures need to be constantly evolving in order to give people the best chance of a good quality of life.

A good understanding of all the issues is forefront in bringing about change and pushing for best practice and new treatments.

This new edition is really welcome in helping to make this happen.

Patients, their families and caregivers can all gain a better insight of kidney disease and its treatment through reading this book, and I recommend it to anyone who wants to learn more about their condition or to re-evaluate the various treatment options.

Patricia Rogers BD MSc FinstF
Chief Executive
National Kidney Federation

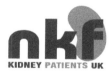

ACKNOWLEDGEMENTS

We are delighted to have this sixth edition of *Kidney Failure Explained* published and recognise that this would not have been possible without the book's original co-author, Dr Andy Stein who wrote the first four editions with Janet. Andy kindly reviewed the final manuscript and we hope he is as proud of this edition as he's been of all the earlier ones.

In addition, we'd like to thank Shanon Rademacher not only for her excellent editing skills but also for her quiet and gentle pestering so that we met our deadlines. Thanks also to our publisher, Dick Warner for believing that this book is worth a sixth edition!

A big thank you also goes to Dr Janson Leung, Consultant Renal Physician who kindly reviewed the chapter on transplantation. His suggestions and comments were very valuable.

We are grateful to 'Think Kidneys' for permission to reproduce the infographic on pages 4–5. We would also like to thank those people who have generously allowed us to use their photographs on the cover of this book. They are all people who know from experience what it is like to live with kidney failure – and yet as the pictures prove they still know how to enjoy many aspects of life. So thanks to Fatima Randera, Michelle Anderson and her boys Oliver and Lewis, Sarah Hirst Williams, Kirsty Hutchinson and her son Alfie, Ameer Basnet and his family, Earnest Wheeler and Marjorie James. Thanks too to Kidney Care UK for providing additional photographs, and Rich Stone for helping to make this cover a reality.

The list of 'thank yous' would not be complete without acknowledging the huge support we have both had from our families.

Janet Wild and Richard Fluck

PREFACE

This is a book about kidney failure and its treatment. It is rare that kidney failure affects only the person who has been given the diagnosis. It affects whole families, friends and work colleagues. The diagnosis can be as devastating for those on the sidelines as it is for the person at the centre. But, for many people, finding out information and learning to understand their illness can help them get to grips with the problems. With this in mind we have written a book that we hope will be useful to anyone affected by kidney failure.

Both authors of this book believe that the more you know about your kidney failure and its treatment, the better you will be able to cope with it. Kidney medicine, along with all medical specialties, is rife with jargon, abbreviations and acronyms. However, once you get through all the specialist terminology, there should be no aspect of healthcare that is too complicated or difficult to explain. In this book, we have set out to dispel the myths, unravel the jargon and explain all matters of the kidney as simply and straightforwardly as possible.

The aim therefore is to give you, the reader, the knowledge and confidence to ask questions. This in turn will make it easier for you to get the right information, phrased in the right way. Then you can use this information to make the choices that are best for you, take control of what happens to you and enjoy your life in spite of your kidney failure.

It has been 20 years since the first edition of this book was published. In this version we've focused more on how you can take control, while also updating the clinical issues, text and keeping it relevant.

We hope that, armed with information, patients and their loved ones, can get the best health for themselves, and work to improve things for others.

Janet Wild and Richard Fluck

SECTION 1:

What do my kidneys do, how do they go wrong and how is kidney failure diagnosed?

1 WHAT IS KIDNEY FAILURE?

This first chapter begins by explaining how kidneys work. Then it explores what goes wrong when someone has established kidney failure, what causes this problem and why it should be treated.

Introduction

Chronic kidney impairment or disease (CKD) is a common and serious problem. It is estimated that one in ten adults have CKD. An individual with CKD has three potential medical risks. First, it may progress to established renal failure. Second, people are at greater risk of heart attack, strokes and other cardiovascular diseases. Third, it increases the risk of a temporary reduction in kidney function - we call this acute kidney injury (AKI).

Chronic kidney disease has many possible causes, but the effects are usually the same. The kidneys become less and less able to do their normal work. After a time, the kidneys may stop working almost completely – a condition known as established renal failure (ERF), end-stage renal disease (ESRD) or end-stage kidney failure. You may hear any one of these names for kidney failure, but the most widely used term now is established renal failure, or ERF.

A small number of people who have CKD will develop kidney failure which will need treatment either with a kidney transplant or with dialysis. At the present time, there are approximately 57,000 people in the UK who are either on dialysis or have received a kidney transplant to treat chronic kidney failure. Of these, 42% are on haemodialysis (1,200 of these have haemodialysis at home), 6% on peritoneal dialysis (PD) and 52% have a transplant. Just over one person in 1,100 has kidney failure, making it a rare condition. This means that a typical family doctor will have only one or two kidney patients 'on their books'.

There are approximately 7,000 new patients diagnosed with ERF each year in the UK. When the kidneys stop working in this way, treatment that takes over the work they do becomes essential. The main treatments are either transplantation or dialysis – either peritoneal dialysis (PD) which is done at home, or haemodialysis (HD) which can be done either in hospital or at home. These treatments cannot 'cure' kidney failure, but they can improve health and prolong life.

Kidneys – what and where are they?

In health the kidneys have several important functions. Not everyone is aware of these complex roles in keeping us well but it is useful to understand them. The kidneys clear the body of toxins, regulate the salt and fluid balance of our bodies, stimulate the production of red blood cells, control our blood pressure and have a role in bone health. The Think Kidneys national project has produced a useful summary of the kidneys in health and illness and with permission it is replicated here.

Most people have two kidneys. These important body organs are shaped like beans and are about 12 centimetres (5 inches) long, which is about the length of a man's palm. They are approximately 6 centimetres wide and

(Almost) everything you need to know about your kidneys

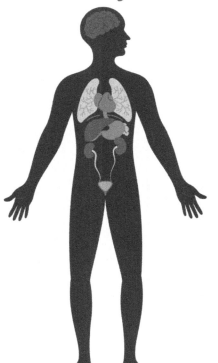

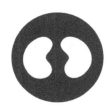

Most people have two kidneys
They are about the size of your clenched fist, they each weigh around 150g and are shaped like kidney beans

They sit in your lower back under the bottom ribs
Only 50% of the population know that kidneys produce urine

They filter your blood every minute of the day
Your blood goes through the kidneys 40 times in 24 hours. There are 140 miles of tubes and a million filters in your kidneys

They are the hardest working organs in your body
They use 25% of the blood from every heartbeat

What do your kidneys do?

┌ Make urine ┐   ┌ Produce hormones ┐   Activate Vitamin D   Clean your blood

Regulate salt and water in your body, making about 3-4 pints of urine each day

Remove waste products from your blood into your urine

Regulate your blood pressure

Create erythropoietin to control the production of red blood cells

Keep bones healthy

Remove many drugs that some people take for other conditions

How to keep your kidneys healthy

┌──────────── Lead a healthy lifestyle ────────────┐

Keep hydrated

Don't smoke

Keep your weight down

Exercise regularly

Eat a healthy diet including fresh fruit, vegetables and fish

Reduce your intake of salt, processed foods and high sugar drinks

If you take regular medication ask your pharmacist how it may affect your kidneys

What causes kidney problems?

One of the most common causes of kidney disease is diabetes

But there are many others including genetic and inflammatory conditions, blockages of urine flow and high blood pressure that can be a cause and/or consequence of kidney problems.

About 1 in 10 people has some form of Chronic Kidney Disease (CKD)

CKD is a long term loss of kidney function which can be harmful. Not all CKD gets worse but it can lead to kidney failure. CKD also increases the risk of heart attack or stroke and increases the risk of acute kidney injury.

Acute Kidney Injury (AKI) is serious and can occur when a person is unwell

AKI is a quick reduction in kidney function. Finding AKI in the early stages is very important as it can make other health problems more difficult to treat.

Of emergency admissions to hospital 1 in 5 people have AKI

AKI can occur after major surgery or with heart problems. Up to 100,000 deaths in hospital in the UK each year are associated with AKI. It causes harm and suffering and costs a lot.

Why you need to think kidneys

If you are worried about your kidneys visit your GP and find out if screening is necessary

Always 'Think Kidneys' when visiting your GP as CKD and AKI often show few symptoms

Your kidneys are remarkable and can look after you at just 10% functionality

AKI often gets better and can even recover fully as the underlying problems are treated

What are the symptoms of kidney problems?

In the early stages of kidney disease there are often no symptoms

There may be no pain or reduction in urine output. Kidney problems are found by a simple blood or urine test so we recommend that people at risk of CKD or AKI are tested regularly to spot problems as soon as possible.

Symptoms of more serious kidney problems can include:

• Tiredness • Frequent headaches • Loss of appetite • Sleep problems • Itchy skin • Nausea or vomiting • Swelling or numbing of the hands or feet • Passing urine more (especially at night) or less often than usual • Darkening / lightening of the skin • Muscle cramps

'THINK KIDNEYS'

Think Kidneys is a national programme led by NHS England in partnership with UK Renal Registry

Kidney disease is serious. It's harmful and changes lives. Protect your kidneys as if your life depended on it: because it does!

Find out how to keep your kidneys healthy and safe www.thinkkidneys.nhs.uk

You can become a donor and help save a life by signing up at: www.organdonation.nhs.uk

Your kidneys are amazing. They work so hard for you. Look after them and Think Kidneys

Figure 1.1: 'Think Kidneys' infographic.

Reproduced with permission.

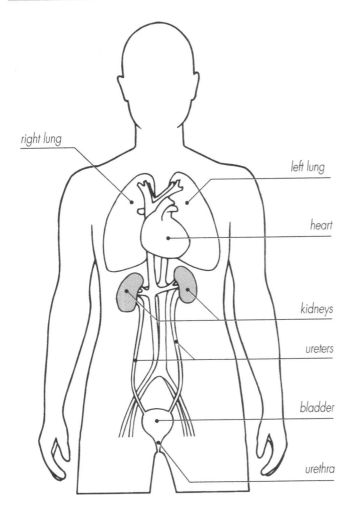

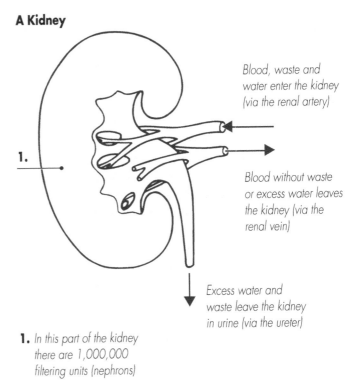

The kidneys' main job: making urine

The main job of the kidneys is to be the body's dustmen. They clean up the blood and use the urine to get rid of the waste products they take out of it. When urine is passed, the rubbish is taken away.

How does this happen? Blood is pumped by the heart to the kidneys. The kidneys have a complex filter system that in health 'cleans' the blood. The urine is made up of water, salts and toxins that are a product of the filter system working on the body's blood. About 180 litres of blood get processed every day – in other words all your blood gets cleaned 30–40 times a day. From that just 2 litres of urine are made each day.

Each kidney has a drainage system that takes urine from that kidney to the bladder. This drainage system is

Figure 1.2: Location of kidneys and urinary system

3 centimetres thick. Each kidney weighs about 150 grams (6 ounces). The kidneys sit under the lower ribs at the back, one on either side of the body (see Figure 1.2). The kidneys lie deep inside the body, so you cannot normally 'feel' them.

A Kidney

Blood, waste and water enter the kidney (via the renal artery)

Blood without waste or excess water leaves the kidney (via the renal vein)

Excess water and waste leave the kidney in urine (via the ureter)

1. In this part of the kidney there are 1,000,000 filtering units (nephrons)

A Kidney filtering unit (nephron)

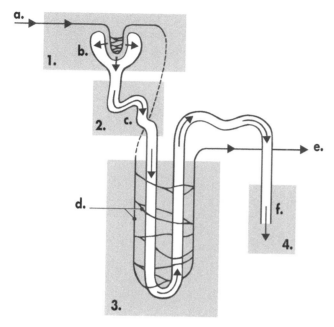

1. *Blood from the renal artery (**a.**) is filtered inside a glomerulus (**b.**).*
2. *Water and waste products filtered from the blood enter a tube system (**c.**).*
3. *Blood vessels (**d.**) take most of the water back around the body via the renal vein (**e.**).*
4. *Waste products and excess water (the urine) are removed via a drainage duct (**f.**) that eventually drains into the bladder.*

Figure 1.3: How the kidney filters blood

like a funnel with a tube (the ureter) that connects the kidney to the bladder (see Figure 1.3). Urine passes down the ureters (one for each kidney) into the bladder. Urine is stored in the bladder before being passed from the body via another tube, called the urethra. The bladder holds about 400 ml (3⁄4 pint) of urine when 'full'. But when you have just emptied it, by going to the toilet, it will be almost completely empty.

Why make urine?

The kidneys make urine in order to perform their two most important functions. These are:

1. Removing excess salt and fluid from the body – a process called 'ultrafiltration'. (See ultrafiltration for a brief description, and Chapter 11 for more details.)
2. Removing wastes from the blood – a process called 'clearance'. (See below for a brief description, and Chapter 3 for more details.)

Removing excess fluid

One of the most important functions of the kidneys is to remove excess salt and water from the body. As well as getting rid of the waste products of food, healthy kidneys also remove excess fluids from the body. Like the food that we eat, the water (and tea, coffee, beer and all other liquids) that we drink is digested in the stomach and bowels and absorbed into the blood. When the blood reaches the kidneys, the normal sieving and filtering process removes any excess fluid and puts it in the urine. So, normal urine contains not only the waste products of food, but also any excess water that has been drunk. In health, the kidneys are able to carefully regulate how much urine it makes – for example, if it's a hot day and you are sweating more, the kidneys will get rid of less fluid. If you have drunk more than usual, more fluid will be removed. The kidneys can also tell whether you need to lose more salt or water (or vice versa) - they are able to regulate the fluid content of our body to keep us well.

When kidneys fail, they are unable to regulate our salt and water balance so well. People with established kidney failure don't usually pass much urine. Excess fluid can therefore build up in the body, causing it to become 'waterlogged' – a condition called fluid overload (see Chapter 11). This will eventually lead to swelling of the ankles, and shortness of breath due to excess fluid in the lungs. But it is important to remember that people with kidney disease (as opposed to kidney failure) will pass normal amounts of urine but are not able to deal with either dehydration or over hydration.

Removing toxic wastes

The kidneys also play a very important role in getting rid of waste products. The food we eat is digested in the stomach and the bowels. During digestion, the food is broken down into substances that can be carried around the body in the blood. These 'good things' in the bloodstream provide every part of the body with the energy it needs to work, and with the substances necessary for growth and repair.

When the different parts of the body make use of the various 'good things' in the blood, they also produce waste products. These wastes are toxic (poisonous) to the body and make people unwell unless they are removed. Like the 'good things', these 'bad things' also travel around the body in the bloodstream.

When the waste products of food in the blood reach the kidneys, it is the job of the kidneys to get rid of them in the urine. What the kidneys do is to sieve and filter the blood, removing the wastes and putting them in the urine, but leaving the 'good things' in the blood. Healthy kidneys generally have no problems getting rid of all the many waste products normally produced by the body.

In people with kidney failure, however, the levels of waste products build up in the blood. It is this build-up of waste products that makes people with kidney failure feel unwell. When someone is in the early stages of kidney failure, there are usually no symptoms, because the levels of waste products are not high enough to cause problems. (This can be true even when the kidneys are working at less than 25% of their normal capacity.)

Other functions of the kidney

As well as fluid and waste removal, the kidneys have three important 'extra' functions. These are:

1   Helping to control blood pressure. The blood pressure is finely controlled by healthy kidneys. When someone's kidneys fail, their blood pressure usually goes up. High blood pressure is unlikely to cause symptoms unless the pressure gets very high, but it increases the risk of a stroke or heart attack, and can cause the kidneys to deteriorate more rapidly (see also Chapter 12).

2   Helping to control the manufacture of red blood cells. The kidneys help control the making of red blood cells in the bone marrow (the runny bit in the middle of all bones). The red blood cells float in the liquid part of the blood (called plasma). Their job is to carry oxygen around the body. Every part of the body needs oxygen to function properly. When someone has kidney failure, they make fewer red blood cells than normal. This causes them to become anaemic (i.e. they are short of red blood cells). This anaemia contributes to the tiredness suffered by most people with kidney failure – it is not only high waste levels that cause tiredness. (See Chapter 7 for more about anaemia and how it can be treated.)

3   Helping to keep the bones strong and healthy. Calcium and phosphate (Chapter 13) are two minerals found in the blood and in the bones. If the bones are to stay strong and healthy, there must be a correct balance between these minerals in the body. The kidneys help to maintain this balance. They do this by activating vitamin D to allow it act on the bones and to get rid of phosphate. When someone develops kidney failure, the normal balance between calcium and phosphate in the body is lost. The level of calcium in the blood goes down, while the level of phosphate in the blood goes up. Unless this imbalance is treated, it will result in a condition called renal bone disease. This may cause aches and pains in the bones, and even fractures. (See Chapter 7 for more information about renal bone disease and its treatment.)

Kidney failure – what is it?

In short, kidney failure is a condition in which the kidneys are less able than normal to perform their usual functions. These functions are:

- removing waste products from the body;
- removing excess water;

- helping to control blood pressure;
- helping to control red blood cell manufacture; and
- helping to keep the bones strong and healthy.

This book is about the long-term condition known as kidney failure and how it can be treated.

There is a separate condition, known as acute kidney failure or acute kidney injury (AKI), in which the kidneys suddenly stop working. Short-term treatment may be needed for AKI, but the kidneys usually get better on their own. This book does not tell you about AKI.

When kidneys start to fail, they become less and less able to do their work. This usually happens gradually over a period of many years. Eventually, the kidneys stop working almost completely. This is when the condition is described as established renal failure or ERF. Treatment is then essential to take over the work of the kidneys and so keep the patient alive. The treatments for ERF are dialysis or a kidney transplant (see Chapters 3 and 6).

What are the symptoms?

In the early stages of chronic kidney disease, there are often no symptoms. Symptoms may develop from the kidney failure itself or from the complications of kidney failure and may result in any of the following:

- itching;
- weakness or tiredness;
- loss of appetite;
- poor concentration;
- restless legs;
- leg cramps;
- swollen ankles;
- shortness of breath;
- poor sleeping;
- low sex drive; and
- feeling cold.

How is kidney failure diagnosed?

Kidney failure is diagnosed by measuring kidney function. This is done by calculating the rate at which the kidneys are able to perform their function of filtering the blood. This is measured in millilitres per minute (a bit like miles per hour but using millilitres of blood instead of miles and minutes instead of hours) and is called the Glomerular Filtration Rate or GFR. Healthy kidneys can filter about 100 millilitres of blood in a minute.

The GFR is estimated using a blood test for a substance called creatinine. Creatinine is produced when your muscles are used and is one of the many waste products that build up in the blood when someone has kidney failure. The level of creatinine is used in a calculation that includes the patient's gender, age and ethnic origin. The GFR result is similar to a percentage of kidney function, so someone who has a GFR of 50 mls/min has 50% kidney function. It is not a completely accurate measurement and so is often referred to as the Estimated GFR or eGFR. There are very accurate ways to measure GFR but they are more cumbersome to use as a routine test.

In addition, a test will be made on the urine to see whether the kidneys are leaking protein. A small sample of urine is used to measure either albumin (one type of protein) or total protein. This is compared to the amount of creatinine in the urine to give an albumin creatinine ratio (urinary ACR) or a protein creatinine ratio (urinary PCR). Normally the kidneys only allow very small amounts of protein to pass through the filter system from blood to urine. Damaged kidneys can leak an excess of protein.

Chronic kidney disease is diagnosed using these two tests – a measurement of eGFR and of how much protein has leaked into the urine, called urine protein excretion. These two tests are used to diagnose, classify and monitor CKD. A single blood or urine test is not enough to determine someone has CKD. At least two tests, three months apart, is recommended by NICE (in NICE Clinical Guideline CG 182: Chronic Kidney Disease in Adults: assessment and management, last updated January 2015). The estimated GFR is then used to provide a stage of CKD and this is used to guide monitoring treatment and planning (see Figure 1.4).

Stage	GFR	Description	Treatment stage
1	90+	Near normal kidney function but urine tests, genetic diseases or scans of the kidney show signs of kidney disease	Observation, control of blood pressure
2	60–89	Mildly reduced kidney function, and other findings (as for Stage 1) point to kidney disease	Observation, control of blood pressure and risk factors
3	44–59	Moderately reduced kidney function	Observation, control of blood pressure and risk factors
4	15–29	Severely reduced kidney function	Planning for established renal failure
5	<15 or on dialysis	Very severe, or established kidney failure	Treatment choices

Figure 1.4: Stages of CKD based on eGFR

eGFR is not only used to detect kidney failure, but also used at all stages of kidney disease – before dialysis and after a transplant. The eGFR is the single most important piece of information that doctors and nurses require when looking after people with kidney failure. (See Chapter 13 for more information.)

If you have kidney failure, you should know what your eGFR is all the time. Ask the nurse or doctor to tell you the value each time you have a blood test or even better, ask your renal unit if you can sign up for 'Patient View' (www.patientview.org) where you can see all of your test results online. More details can be found in Chapter 2. It can be useful to look at the progress of your kidney failure by plotting the eGFR on a graph so that you can see, over time, how quickly or slowly your kidneys are failing. Patient View does this for you.

The 'progression' of kidney failure

When chronic kidney failure is still at an early stage, most patients feel quite well. This is because their failing kidneys 'overwork' to keep the level of body waste normal. This hides the fact that the kidneys are failing.

In other words, the kidneys have a lot 'in reserve'. The body manages for quite some time to adapt to high levels of waste products and excess water in the blood. It does this by making the kidneys work harder. The rate at which kidney disease gets worse varies from patient to patient. Also, the symptoms that patients get when they have similar levels of kidney function can vary considerably.

However, for most people, the stages of their kidney disease will be as shown in the table above. The vast majority of people who have Stages 1, 2 and 3 do not progress to ERF. However, if you are reading this book it is likely that you or someone you care about has Stage 4 kidney disease or worse and may develop kidney failure in the future.

What causes kidneys to fail?

There are hundreds of different diseases that can cause kidneys to start failing, and sometimes to fail completely. Usually, however, ERF (leading to dialysis or a transplant) is likely to be due to one of the following causes:

1 **Diabetes mellitus.** Diabetes is the most common known cause of kidney failure in the developed

world where it may be the cause of ERF in up to 40% of patients in some countries. Whether diabetes is controlled by insulin, tablets or diet, it can cause kidney failure (known as diabetic nephropathy). This is more likely to happen when someone has had diabetes for more than 10 years. In the UK, an average of 25% of new dialysis patients every year are thought to be suffering from diabetic nephropathy.

2   **Nephritis.** The term 'nephritis' means inflammation of the kidneys ('nephr-' indicates 'kidney', and 'itis' means 'inflammation'). The term is usually applied to people with glomerulonephritis or GN. ('Glomerulo' refers to the glomeruli, which are part of the kidneys' filtration unit.)

The causes of most types of nephritis are unknown. Nephritis is another condition that can only be diagnosed for certain by a kidney biopsy.

3   **Autosomal Dominant Polycystic Kidney Disease (ADPKD).** This is an inherited disease (a disease that runs in families) in which both kidneys become filled ('poly' means 'many') with cysts (abnormal fluid-filled lumps). If someone has ADPKD, they will have a 50% chance of passing the condition on to each of their children. The problem is diagnosed by ultrasound (an investigation that uses sound waves to produce a picture of the kidneys) and from family history. Polycystic kidneys, although abnormally large because of the cysts, do not work well and many people eventually develop ERF.

The cysts in PKD can remain a problem after treatment for kidney failure has started. A cyst can burst, bleed or get infected – any of which may cause pain. Sometimes, people with polycystic kidneys have to have one or both kidneys removed to make room for a transplanted kidney.

Further information can be found at the PKD charity website – http://pkdcharity.org.uk.

4   **Pyelonephritis.** 'Pyelo' (meaning 'funnel') refers to the drainage system of the kidney and 'nephritis' means 'kidney inflammation', so pyelonephritis means 'inflammation of the kidney drainage system'. Pyelonephritis is diagnosed by ultrasound, or by a special X-ray of the kidneys called an intravenous pyelogram (IVP), in which an opaque dye is injected into the bloodstream. It can also be diagnosed by a special nuclear medicine scan of the kidneys (called a DMSA or MAG-3 scan), in which a small amount of a radioactive substance is injected into the bloodstream.

Pyelonephritis can sometimes be linked to repeated kidney infections. These may have gone undetected for many years, perhaps having occurred in childhood. Pyelonephritis is sometimes caused by a condition called reflux nephropathy (or 'reflux'). In this condition, a valve where the ureter enters the bladder (see Figure 1.5) is faulty. This faulty valve allows urine from the bladder to flow back up the ureter to cause problems in the kidney. Reflux is a partially inherited condition, particularly in women. So the children of patients with reflux should be tested for it soon after birth. This is true for boys and girls, whichever parent has the condition.

5   **Renovascular disease.** As people get older, their arteries tend to become 'furred' up with cholesterol and other fats. Diabetes and smoking make this process occur at a younger age. This 'furring up' (which is called atheroma or atherosclerosis) gradually narrows the arteries (the blood vessels that take blood from the heart to every part of the body).

Atheroma in the arteries that supply the heart's own muscle leads to angina and heart attacks. If the atheroma affects the arteries that supply blood to the brain, it may cause a stroke. Atheroma can also affect and block the arteries that supply blood to the kidneys, the renal arteries. This is called renovascular disease ('reno' means kidney, and 'vascular' means blood vessel). Renovascular disease is a particularly common cause of kidney failure in older patients. A renal angiogram is the only way of definitely diagnosing the condition. But this procedure carries some risk, so it is not done routinely for every patient.

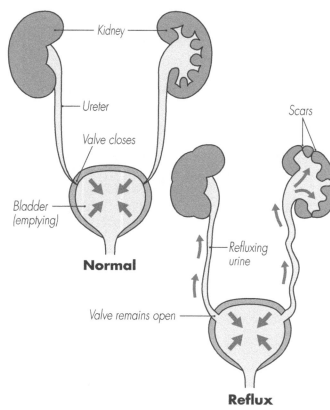

Figure 1.5: What happens in reflux nephropathy

6 **Obstructive nephropathy.** This is a common cause of ERF in men, especially those over the age of 60 years. It is usually due to enlargement of the prostate gland, which obstructs the urethra (hence the name 'obstructive nephropathy'). The urethra is the tube through which the urine drains from the bladder. It can also be caused by tumours in the bladder or in the pelvis. There are other causes in both men and women.

Relieving the blockage can often reverse the kidney failure. But in some people, especially those who were diagnosed late, ERF requiring dialysis or a transplant will occur, even if the patient has had an operation on the prostate to relieve the blockage.

7 **Unknown.** In about 14% of patients with ERF, the cause of the kidney failure is never discovered. This is because the kidneys often appear small and shrunken when shown by ultrasound. For this reason, a diagnosis of 'two small kidneys' is often made. 'Two small kidneys' really means that the kidneys are small, but doctors don't know why. It is presumed that 'something' happened to the kidneys years ago, and they have slowly shrivelled up since.

How is ERF treated?

ERF can be treated by dialysis or by a kidney transplant. Dialysis and transplantation provide alternative ways of taking over the work of the patient's failed kidneys although neither is a cure for kidney failure.

Can the need for dialysis or a transplant be delayed?

Once a patient has developed ERF, treatment should be started very soon. However, if someone with chronic kidney disease has not yet developed ERF, it may be possible to delay the need for dialysis or a transplant. This is particularly true for Stages 1, 2 and 3 of kidney disease, which can often be held 'in check' for years so the patient never progresses to Stage 4 or beyond.

The following treatments may delay the need for dialysis or a transplant in some patients:

1 **Treatments to control blood pressure.** High blood pressure is known to speed up kidney failure. Doctors therefore make great efforts to keep the blood pressure of their kidney patients low. Keeping the blood pressure low (consistently 130/80 mmHg or less) can delay the need for dialysis by years. This is true for most patients with kidney failure – the cause of the kidney failure makes no difference. (See Chapter 12 for more about blood pressure and kidney failure.)

2 **Treatments to slow down the underlying kidney disease.** When kidney failure is due to nephritis, the need for dialysis can sometimes be delayed by tablets called immunosuppressants. In some types of nephritis, the body's immune system (the system that normally fights infection or foreign objects in the body) starts to attack the patient's kidneys and stops them working properly. So tablets that make the immune system less effective – such as the steroid tablet called prednisolone – can be used to treat the kidney problem. In some patients, such treatments are very successful, and return the kidney function to normal or near normal. In other patients, these tablets are less successful. Even so, they may delay the need for dialysis or a transplant by many years. (There is more information on the immune system in Chapter 6.)

3 **Use of ACE inhibitors/angiotensin receptor blockers (ARBs).** Some people with kidney failure (especially kidney failure caused by diabetes or nephritis) have a large amount of protein in the urine. Blood pressure tablets called 'ACE inhibitors' (e.g. lisinopril) or ARBs (e.g. irbesartan) are often used by kidney doctors to treat high blood pressure in people with CKD especially if they have raised protein levels in the urine. Some research studies have shown that this will slow down the progression of kidney failure. Using these types of blood pressure tablets is recommended by NICE (see Chapter 14 for more information about NICE).

4 **Treating obstructive nephropathy.** This is done either by putting a plastic tube (urinary catheter) into the bladder through the urethra; or one or more tubes (nephrostomies) through the skin, into the pelvis (drainage system) of the kidney. Depending on the cause of the obstruction, these procedures in men are usually followed by an operation on the prostate gland, after which the plastic tubes can usually be taken out. Women do not have a prostate gland, so obstruction in a woman would be caused by something else.

Will dialysis or a transplant solve the problem?

Neither dialysis nor a kidney transplant can 'cure' a patient with ERF. These treatments can control the symptoms of kidney failure, but they cannot get rid of the symptoms completely nor restore the kidneys to health.

KEY FACTS

1 The two main functions of your kidneys are:
   a removing excess water and salt
   b removing waste products.

2 They also control your blood pressure, stimulate your bone marrow to produce red blood cells and are vital for bone health.

3 If your kidneys are impaired or failing, they will be less able to carry out these functions.

4 Whatever the original cause of your kidney failure, it is likely to get worse over a period of years.

5 A simple blood and urine test is used to diagnose and monitor the progression of kidney disease. A test (the GFR) is used to measure the amount of work that the kidneys can still do. This is normally about 100 mls/min, equivalent to 100% of kidney function. If it is less than 60 mls/min (i.e. 60%) you have kidney impairment.

6 People with chronic (Stage 4) kidney disease (eGFR <30 mls/min, i.e. <30%) have the highest risk to develop ERF, when they will need dialysis or a transplant.

7 For most kidney patients, good control of blood pressure is essential to delay the onset of ERF and the need for dialysis.

SECTION 2:

What treatments are available, and how will kidney failure affect my daily life?

2 TAKING CONTROL FROM THE START

In this chapter we explain what you can do to take control of your kidney failure and general health. Being involved with your own care and sharing the responsibility with your healthcare professionals will help you to feel better both physically and emotionally.

Introduction

Having a good understanding of your kidney problems, what causes them and how they are treated is very important. People who develop their knowledge, acquire the right skills to look after themselves and are more confident about their own healthcare often feel much more in control and tend to be happier. It is also more likely that having a better understanding of your health will help you to make better choices about your health treatments and manage your condition more effectively.

Knowing about the treatments that are available

Developing your knowledge and understanding of the different treatments that are available is very important. When someone has kidney failure there are lots of different treatments: dialysis and transplants, treatments for high blood pressure, anaemia, bone problems and for other symptoms you may experience. Understanding what each treatment does and what the benefits or possible problems are can help in very many ways.

Building your knowledge

Knowing and understanding about your kidney disease and its treatments is the first step towards taking control.

There are very many places that you can learn – reading this book is an obvious first choice, for example.

The internet. There is plenty of information available on the internet; however, it is important to remember that the information on some websites is not always reliable or accurate. It is always a good idea to ask your healthcare team which websites they would recommend. You can check at the back of this book for some useful websites that you might want to explore.

Your team. The team of doctors, nurses, dietitians and other healthcare professionals at the renal unit are an excellent source of information. They often have years of experience looking after people with kidney failure and so will be able to answer your questions. Remember that looking after your health is a team effort. The team includes you and your family, as well as the people at the hospital.

Some good opportunities for you to build your knowledge are explained below.

Other patients, family members or members of the public. One of the most powerful sources of advice and information is other patients. It might be an informal chat with someone in the waiting room or on the ward. It may be as part of an education day where experienced patients are asked to speak, or it may be from a trained 'peer-support' patient. We know that you will listen to them and their experience very closely because they will be giving you insider knowledge. However, we would always recommend speaking to more than one patient and their family to get a better understanding. It is always a good idea to ask your renal team whether they can help. If you have come away with a strong view about something – it might be about a tablet, or a type of treatment – remember to discuss it with your renal team. What has or hasn't worked for one person may not be the full story, so it is important to be able to put that in context. Do listen to people who have experience of what you are going through but remember one size doesn't fit all!

Clinic visits. Take the opportunity at clinic visits to ask questions about things that you don't understand or that have been worrying you. It's a good idea to prepare for meetings with the doctors and other members of the team. Think about what you want to talk about and write down a list of the things you want to discuss. There might not always be a lot of time available with the doctor during the clinic visit. Ask before you go how much time you have and then prioritise the questions to make sure that you have the chance to ask the most important ones.

Often, the Specialist Nurses have more time to spend with patients, so it's worth asking if you can have a special meeting with one of them. Don't forget that the dietitian is also a great source of information, and planning for these meetings is equally important. Some units may also have a pharmacist or a physiotherapist available to help with other queries. Find out who is in the clinic you attend and whether other members of the team are available for you to see.

Don't be shy about bringing a friend or relative along to the clinic with you. It is often helpful to have two pairs of ears to listen to what's being said. They may also think of other questions that may not have occurred to you.

Letters to your family doctor/GP. After each clinic visit, the doctor will write a letter to your family doctor explaining what was discussed and your treatment plan. Ask if you can have a copy of this letter so you have a record. There may be things in the letter that you have forgotten about, or that you didn't fully understand.

Some kidney doctors address these letters to the patient rather than the GP, or write to both of you. This is an excellent idea as it encourages the doctor to write in a language that patients can more easily understand. Why not ask your doctor if it is possible to write to you and send a copy of the letter to your GP?

Patient information events. Many hospitals run events during the evening or the daytime for patients and their relatives or friends. These sessions can be very helpful to give you more detail about the treatments available. There are often many other patients attending and you will have the opportunity to talk to others in a similar position to yourself. Sometimes, patients who are already on dialysis or who have a transplant go to these events to share their experiences.

Patient View

Patient View (often known as PV) is an excellent tool to help you to become more involved in your treatment and care. It is a website that is designed to be used by both patients and the renal unit to keep a record of your test results, medicines and other information. It works by taking information from your electronic record at the hospital, from the system used by the renal unit, and presents the data on a web portal. It is very secure and each patient has a user name and password which gives them access to their personal information. This password can be shared with family members if you want, but it is your information.

All the Renal Centres in England are required to offer Patient View to patients. So, when you have a clinic appointment with the kidney doctor, ask about it and find out how you can sign up to get your log in details so that you can have access to the site.

The site is divided into the following sections:

My Details. This is where your personal details are recorded such as your name, date of birth, address and phone number and your GP contact details. This section of the site also has space for you to write down the things you would like your healthcare team to know about you, for example your interests, if you have caring responsibilities for someone else or grandchildren, if you travel frequently, work or have other commitments that you think the doctors and nurses should know about. There is also space in this section for you to make a note of things you'd like to talk about – for example questions about the progression of your kidney failure, your treatment or decisions you have made.

The nurses and doctors have access to the information so will be able to read anything you write here. You can use this for discussions at clinic visits.

My Condition. This is where your diagnosis and other conditions are recorded. This section of the site also contains links to further information about kidney problems, treatments for kidney failure and some decision making tools. This part of PV will also display your 'transplant status'. This will show you if you are on the list for a kidney transplant or not, are suspended from the list (perhaps because you have a temporary health problem, or because you are away, or maybe because the results of some tests haven't yet been received), or if you have a transplant.

Results. This is the main part of the site where your test results are uploaded and stored. All of your blood and other test results are here, including your blood pressure, height and weight. The results can be viewed as the most recent result or as a graph so that you can see how they have changed over time. This is useful, particularly for your eGFR before you start treatment, as it can show you the progression of your kidney failure. (See Chapter 1 for more detail.)

You can also use the site to store your blood pressure, weight and blood sugars if you have diabetes. It's a good idea to use this site to record these on a regular basis. The team at the renal unit can then use this information if they need it to help them make decisions about your treatments. It's also valuable to have a record of blood pressure and weight changes over time.

Medicines. A list of all the medicines that you take is part of your hospital record and will be on the PV system. However, it's a good idea to check that the list on PV has the same medicines that you take. Let your doctor or nurse know if you think there are any mistakes or if anything has changed when you have seen your GP or another doctor. There is a link on this section that takes you to another site that will give more information about the medicines you are taking, if you would like more detail.

Letters. A record of all the letters that have been written to you or your GP can be stored on this section of the site. Letters are only stored if they are on the renal unit's computer system that links to PV, so it might not be complete.

Contact Details. This is a list of all useful addresses and phone numbers for the different departments at your own renal unit.

Keeping records yourself

Taking part in your care means that you will be asked to keep a record of your health.

Blood pressure recording. Blood pressure machines are not expensive and are widely available from high street chemists but make sure you get an approved model. The British Hypertension Society (bhsoc.org) has a list of ones they have tested. Get one that uses a cuff that goes around your upper arm, **not** one that goes around the wrist – you may need to check you get the right size cuff as well. They also need looking after – ask your supplier how to do that but they should be checked every two years. They are easy to use, but the nurses at the hospital or at your GP practice will be very happy to give you a lesson in 'taking your own blood pressure'.

People are often more relaxed at home than they are when visiting the hospital, so blood pressure recordings from home are likely to be more accurate. Also, having a blood pressure machine at home will allow you to take recordings frequently over a period of time. This can give the doctors and nurses good information about how well your condition is being managed, how well the tablets are working or if you need to start taking or change your blood pressure tablets.

Ask how often you need to check your blood pressure – in most cases once a week is more than enough.

Weight. Keeping a record of your weight is a good idea for a number of reasons. Your weight can be a useful guide to how much fluid you have in your body (see Chapter 11 for more details). As your kidney function gets worse, you may stop passing as much urine as normal which can lead to fluid retention. Sometimes this is difficult to spot, but if your weight has increased suddenly, it may show that you have too much fluid in your body.

Some people who have kidney failure may feel sick and have a poor appetite. Keeping a record of your weight is useful to find out if you have lost weight. Losing weight may make some of your blood test results slightly inaccurate, so it's always helpful to bear in mind weight loss when looking at blood results. Equally, being overweight can affect your kidney function, increase your risk of heart problems and reduce the chances of a successful transplant.

Remember, you can record your blood pressure and your weight on Patient View if you have access to the internet.

Nutrition. Some people will also take nutritional supplements such as multivitamins. You may also be offered food supplements or drinks that are high in energy or protein. These can be helpful if you are not able to eat much. Keeping a record of what you have taken is a good idea.

Understanding your medicines

People who have kidney failure usually have to take very many different medicines. It is important to know what each medicine is for, how often you need to take it, what to do if you forget a dose and how to order more supplies.

Knowing about your drugs can help you to make decisions about your treatment and prevent problems. For example, if you are taking tablets for high blood pressure, and you notice that your blood pressure has gone down, you can talk to the doctor about the need to take the tablets.

Most people with kidney failure will take tablets for the following conditions:

Blood pressure. These drugs are called 'anti-hypertensives'.

Anaemia. There are two types of treatment for anaemia:
- Iron supplements which are usually taken as tablets, but may also be given as an intravenous infusion (a drip).
- Erythropoetin Stimulating Agents or ESAs. These are usually given as injections.

Bone problems. There are two groups of treatment for bone problems. First, you may take tablets to provide you with 'activated' vitamin D (e.g. One alpha) or to lower a hormone called parathyroid hormone (PTH) – cinacalcet. Then most people on dialysis need drugs to help remove a substance called phosphate from their diet. These also prevent bone problems and are tablets taken with meals. They go under the heading of 'Phosphate Binders' – examples include calcichew, Renagel or Lanthanum.

More information about treatments for bones, anaemia and blood pressure can be found in Chapter 7.

Transplants. Following a kidney transplant you will need to take a number of different medicines to make sure that your body does not 'reject' the new kidney. More information about medication and kidney transplants can be found in Chapter 6.

If you think that you have side effects from taking any of your medicines, it is important to talk to the doctors. There may be alternatives available, or it may be possible for you to stop taking some medicines.

Looking after yourself

A diagnosis of kidney failure has a massive impact. It will affect the whole of your life, not just your physical condition. Once you know you have kidney failure, you will have to make changes to the way you live. You are also likely to find the illness affects the way you feel about yourself, and your priorities in life.

Despite this, it is important to continue to look after your general health by making sure you eat well, take regular exercise and if you smoke, stop.

Advice from the dietitian will be useful to help you to understand how you can eat a healthy diet, even if there are some foods that you need to limit. In addition, it is best to avoid fatty or sugary foods because these can cause obesity or lead to diabetes.

If you are overweight, along with eating more healthily, it's also a good idea to take regular exercise. This doesn't have to involve joining a gym, or training for a marathon. Doing things such as taking regular walks, going swimming or walking up the stairs instead of taking the lift or escalator can all improve your fitness. Keep a record of your physical activity so that you can see how much progress you are making. (More information about diet and exercise can be found in Chapter 8.)

Smoking cigarettes, a pipe or cigars is known to be very harmful. Smoking causes cancer, but it also damages the blood vessels and this in turn can damage the kidneys. So smoking may make your kidney failure worse, or make your kidneys fail sooner. It is very important, therefore, to try to stop smoking.

You can get advice about stopping smoking from your GP or the nurses in the renal unit.

No one expects you to become and expert overnight or do all of these things straight away. But you can build up your confidence gradually, read about your condition to learn more and that will give you the skills you need. Your team want the best for you and the people we see doing well are those that really take control.

KEY FACTS

1 Understanding your health problems, the treatments and taking control will help you feel much better, both physically and emotionally.

2 There are lots of places where you can get information about your health and how kidney disease is treated. Books, the internet and other patients are all good; however it's important to discuss what you've learnt with your healthcare team at the renal centre.

3 Patient View is a website that stores all your personal health information such as blood test results. All English renal units have to offer patients access to this website, so ask when you see your doctor.

4 Monitoring your own health helps you stay in control. You can take and record your own blood pressure and weight and report any concerns to the doctors and nurses at the renal unit.

5 It's important to understand all of the different medicines you take, what they are used for and how to order more if you run out.

6 Looking after your general health is very important. Try to eat well and take lots of exercise. And if you smoke – stop!

3 INTRODUCTION TO DIALYSIS

This chapter describes what dialysis is, how it works and explains how it may fit into your life. It also discusses how patients and carers can take part in their dialysis, either in the hospital renal unit or at home.

Introduction

This is the first of four chapters which explain the treatment options available to people with kidney failure. There are two ways of treating kidney failure: a kidney transplant or dialysis. There is currently no cure. In other words, dialysis or a kidney transplant can replace some of the functions of the kidneys but does not get rid of the kidney disease. Kidney doctors will still consider that you have kidney impairment or failure, whether you are pre-dialysis, on dialysis or have a kidney transplant.

What is dialysis?

Dialysis is an artificial way of doing some of the work of the kidneys. It removes waste products and balances the chemicals in the blood, and it also removes excess water from your body from food and drink.

Almost everyone who has kidney failure will need to have dialysis during their lifetime. Even though many people have a kidney transplant not everyone is suitable for one. Even for those who are, there may not be a suitable kidney immediately available. Also, a kidney transplant does not usually last for a lifetime so dialysis may be needed if a transplant fails.

There are two different types of dialysis: peritoneal dialysis (also called PD, which is done at home), and haemodialysis (also called HD, which can be done at home or in the renal unit).

A brief overview of HD and PD – similarities and differences

PD and HD work in similar ways:

- Waste products are cleared from the blood and the chemicals are brought into balance by a process called diffusion.
- Excess water is removed from the blood by a process known as ultrafiltration.
- Wastes and water pass into a special liquid called the dialysis fluid or dialysate so that they can easily be removed from the body.
- The dialysis actually takes place through a thin layer, known as the dialysis membrane, which keeps the dialysis fluid and blood from mixing together. This membrane has tiny holes which means it can act like a sieve, keeping the important parts of blood but allowing water and wastes to pass across it.

In PD dialysis fluid sits inside the tummy and the membrane is the lining of the tummy. This membrane is called the peritoneum. PD is normally done every day. The process consists of the following three stages:

1   The peritoneal cavity (the part of the tummy where the bowels and other organs are) is filled with about 2 litres of dialysis fluid from a dialysis bag through a small flexible tube which is placed permanently into the abdomen. The amount and type of fluid used can be changed, depending on a patient's individual needs.

2   The dialysis fluid is left inside the peritoneal cavity to allow dialysis to take place. The length of time it stays there varies, from 2 to 8 hours, again depending on individual needs and the type of PD.

3   The 'used' dialysis fluid, containing the water and waste products that the kidneys would normally have removed and passed into the urine, is drained out of the body and is thrown away, usually down the toilet.

In PD, dialysis is happening all the time. This is because the dialysis fluid is always in contact with the dialysis membrane. PD can be done by hand (CAPD) or by using a machine (APD). For more details see Chapter 4.

Haemodialysis works in a similar way, but a man-made membrane is used and blood is pumped out of the body and across the membrane. At the same time dialysis fluid is pumped across the other side of the membrane.

The process of haemodialysis has the following three steps:

1   You are connected to a dialysis machine to allow your blood to be removed (a little at a time) from the body.

2   The blood goes to the dialysis membrane (also called a dialyser) on the machine. At the same time dialysis fluid is pumped by the machine across the other side of the membrane. This is done for relatively short periods of time. For example, if you have haemodialysis in a renal unit, it's normally done for about four hours three times a week. If it's done at home, it can be done more often; either on alternate days, every day for fewer hours, or overnight.

3   Once the treatment is finished you are disconnected from the machine.

PD and three-times-a-week HD provide similar amounts of dialysis (about 5–10% of the function of two healthy kidneys) and this is enough to ease many of the symptoms of kidney failure. However, HD can be done more frequently or for longer, providing more 'dialysis'. Many patients who do frequent HD say that they feel much better, have no symptoms and are not restricted with how much they can eat and drink. In fact, some research that has been done to compare HD three times a week with more frequent HD shows that it is much more effective.

The easiest way to do more HD is to have it at home. This is because you don't need to stick to the renal unit's schedule and can fit the HD sessions in to suit your life.

Starting dialysis – which one first?

Making choices about the treatments for kidney failure is complicated and daunting for everyone. Ideally these choices need thought and time but being involved and in charge of your own decisions generally results in better choices for you and your family. So don't be afraid to ask questions, even difficult ones. Also remember that most people use each type of dialysis during their lifetime as circumstances change. This chapter focuses on the choices between the different ways to do dialysis but there are decisions to be made about kidney transplants or choosing not having any treatment as well.

It is important to think about the long term, in addition to how dialysis will affect your life right now, when deciding on which sort of dialysis to have first. So the order in which you have each type of dialysis can be important to get the best quality of life and the most health benefit. For example, there is evidence that shows having PD as your first treatment has benefits.

Why is that?

Doing PD when your kidneys are still working a little bit can keep them going for longer. In other words, PD is better at preserving the remaining function of your kidneys than HD. That is important for your well-being since this residual kidney function can help fluid balance and waste removal.

The other advantage of doing PD as the first treatment is that you don't need to take blood from the body to do the dialysis. It uses the peritoneum as a natural membrane. This means that you can preserve your blood vessels in case you need to have haemodialysis in the future.

PD is also a home-based treatment that you can do for yourself. So choosing it as a first treatment will mean that you can manage your own dialysis and fit it into your life much more easily than travelling to the hospital three times a week for HD.

If you are worried about looking after yourself at home, there is help available. The nurses will make sure that you are fully trained and confident before you have to do your dialysis yourself. They are always available on the phone too. It usually takes a few days to learn the treatment and the nurses can teach you at home, or in hospital. If you find it difficult to manage alone, healthcare assistants can do some of the dialysis for you, until you become more confident.

Having haemodialysis as a first treatment is also possible if you make that choice. You can either do it in the hospital or be trained to do it at home. Training for home haemodialysis may take a little longer than for PD, depending on the type of machine that is used. Training usually takes place in the haemodialysis unit. You will also need to learn how to put the needles into your arm for dialysis. Most people find that quite daunting but remember that the doctors and nurses looking after you felt the same when they were training. Some people pick this up quickly but others may take a little longer.

When you first start on haemodialysis in hospital, the nurses will help with everything and there is no pressure for you to get involved until you feel ready. But more and more people are now taking part in their treatment and learning about it in more detail.

Dialysis at home or in hospital?

It's important to think about where you would prefer to have your treatment when making a decision about the type of dialysis; at home or in hospital. Both forms of dialysis are effective and most people are suitable for either PD or HD.

It is possible to swap from one type of dialysis to another. In fact many patients will have both PD and HD during their life with kidney failure.

PD is done at home (or anywhere there is a clean and convenient place) whereas HD can be done either at home or in a dialysis unit.

When choosing where to have dialysis, think about:

- **Where you would like to have dialysis.** You can have dialysis at home or in a clinic or hospital. If you decide to have dialysis at home, you will be looked after by a team of people who are dedicated to supporting patients at home on dialysis.
- **How much of the dialysis you would like to do for yourself.** You can get as involved as you like with the dialysis treatment. This is true if you have your dialysis in hospital or at home. It is possible to do some or all of the dialysis for yourself, even if you have the treatment in hospital. Most people who have dialysis at home do the dialysis themselves, but there is also support available for people who can't manage everything.
- **If you would like the dialysis to be able to fit around your life.** Having dialysis in the renal unit usually means that patients have fixed treatment appointments three times a week for four hours each. This enables patients to have four days 'off' dialysis every week. Dialysis at home is more flexible, but is done more frequently. PD is normally undertaken every day and HD can be done between three and seven times per week at home. In addition, both PD and Home HD can be done overnight, leaving day times free for work, study, family and social life. Renal unit-based HD is not as flexible. But in some dialysis units it can be done overnight or in the evening.

- **Would you like to continue to work or go back to work?** Many patients are able to continue to work. Fixed dialysis schedules in hospital can be altered to accommodate work patterns; however those on home-based dialysis usually find it easier to continue their employment. The nurses at the dialysis unit will be happy to speak to a patient's employer about working while on dialysis.
- **If you decide to have your dialysis in the unit, how will you travel to the dialysis unit?** People who have dialysis 'in-centre' at the main renal or a satellite unit will need to make arrangements to get to the unit three times a week. It may be possible for transport to be provided by the hospital, or you might be able to make your own way there. Whatever method of transport is chosen, the time taken to travel to and from the dialysis centre should be taken into account as well as waiting in the unit to start your treatment. Sadly, hospital transport is not always reliable or there can be problems with your treatment that delay you heading home. This can mean that having hospital based dialysis takes up most of the day.
- **If you decide to have dialysis at home, where you will store the supplies?** Dialysis at home requires space to store supplies. Most home dialysis patients will need to store about one month's supplies. The equipment can be stored in the garage, a shed, in the cupboard under the stairs or a spare room. Space also needs to be set aside for the dialysis to be performed. This may need to be in the bedroom if night-time dialysis is chosen.
- **Do you still want to go on holidays and travel?** It is possible to have dialysis away from home. PD patients can have their supplies delivered to their destination. Although this requires forward planning, travel for holidays, family events or business can usually be arranged to most parts of the world within a few weeks (or days in an emergency). More planning is usually required for haemodialysis patients as they need to find a centre in which they can have their treatment while they are away from home. The renal unit will help with the arrangements for both haemodialysis and PD patients to have dialysis away from home.
- **How much contact would you like with other patients?** People who have HD in the renal unit have regular contact with other patients each time they attend for treatment. People on home-based treatments will meet patients if they attend clinics, patient groups or are admitted to hospital.
- **How much contact would you like with healthcare professionals?** Having HD in the renal unit means that there are nurses nearby during each dialysis session. People who have dialysis at home will have regular contact with nurses during home visits, by telephone and at regular clinic visits. Some home dialysis machines have a secure connection to the internet so that the doctors and nurses can keep an eye on your treatment. This means that they can spot problems and deal with them before they get too serious. Some machines also allow the nurses and doctors to update the settings on your machine remotely. This saves them time talking the patient through the process over the phone, or even having to visit the patient at home. This can give patients a lot of reassurance. Everyone who has home dialysis will be trained and educated about all aspects of their treatment. It's a good idea to include a family member or close friend in the training. They can provide support once you get home. Some people who have dialysis at home can have daily assistance from a carer. This might be a paid carer, a relative or partner.

Dialysis and independence

Taking part in your dialysis can have a really positive impact on your life. People who do more for themselves tend to feel more confident, have fewer symptoms and feel more in control. Having said that, it is up to each individual how much they feel happy to do. Some patients may want to look after themselves right from the start, whereas other people may need more support, particularly in the early days.

Discuss the options with the nurses and doctors at the renal unit. Starting the discussion in good time means there is the opportunity to weigh up the pros and cons of each treatment and how you want to be involved. Write a list, using the headings above, take a friend or relative along and talk to your team. They can help you to understand what is involved with each of the treatments.

Making a decision about which type of dialysis

Deciding on a dialysis option can be difficult. However, it is important to remember that you can change your mind and swap between treatments if the one you choose doesn't suit you. As your life changes you may want to change the type of treatment you have. It is really important to make your wishes known to the doctors and nurses in hospital.

It is likely that you would prefer not to have to make a choice at all, as having any type of dialysis is not pleasant. However, there is a lot of support available to help you to make a good decision. A good decision is one that you feel comfortable with once everything has settled down.

People who have been involved in the decision making process tend to feel better about their choice, particularly if they have had enough information to help them make that decision.

One of the kidney charities, Kidney Research UK, has developed a tool to help you, your family and your healthcare team to make the best decision. The 'Dialysis Decision Aid' is available from their website or from your hospital. Ask the nurses or doctors for more information.

Choosing not to have any treatment

When the need for dialysis approaches, those who are elderly, or whose lives are seriously restricted by other illnesses, may decide that they would rather allow nature to 'take its course' – even though this means they will die. There can be some confusion though – in general these conversations and decisions are about planning for the future, not for right now. Advance planning is the key.

It is important for patients and their families to understand that having treatment with a transplant or dialysis is not compulsory. If you do not wish to receive treatment, or decide that you wish to stop dialysis, you should discuss this with the staff at your renal unit. Not having dialysis treatment will mean that the patient will die, usually within a few days or weeks, depending on their degree of kidney failure.

Patients and their families are the only people that can judge whether quality of life with dialysis is acceptable for them but the team as a whole are there to offer their expertise and advice – to support and share in this important decision.

You may be frail or elderly, severely disabled or restricted, yet satisfied that life is still worthwhile.

Teams in the renal unit have a sympathetic attitude and will offer you all the information and support you need in taking this decision. Many renal units now operate a structured conservative care programme. This enables patients who opt not to have dialysis or a transplant to be cared for by the doctors and nurses at their renal unit. They will have the progression of their kidney failure measured and if they experience any symptoms, these can be controlled with medicines.

There may be good medical reasons to decide not to have dialysis, without even considering a trial of treatment. If a patient with kidney failure is already suffering from another terminal illness, for example an inoperable cancer, a progressive brain or blood vessel disease (such as recurrent strokes) or severe heart failure, it can be a relief to be offered the opportunity of refusing dialysis. This can allow a dignified death, in less distressing circumstances than might otherwise apply.

KEY FACTS

1 Dialysis is the word used to describe the removal of body wastes and fluid from the blood.

2 There are two types of dialysis: haemodialysis (HD) and peritoneal dialysis (PD). Both work in a similar way.

3 PD is done in the home setting whereas HD can be done at home or in a hospital or satellite (local) unit

4 Most patients can have either type of dialysis, and may well experience PD and HD at different times.

5 Dialysis removes the body wastes, excess chemicals, and the excess water from the body when the kidneys can't do their job properly.

6 Making the decision about which dialysis to have can be hard. It is important to think about what is best for the long term and it is possible to change treatments from time to time.

7 Taking part in some or all of your dialysis is a positive step. People who are more involved in their care tend to feel better and have fewer symptoms.

8 You can take part in your treatment if you have it in hospital, in a satellite clinic or at home.

9 If you can't manage all the dialysis yourself there are people to support you, either in the hospital or at home.

10 There is always the option of not having any treatment; either dialysis or a transplant. This needs careful consideration as this means that the patient will die within a few days or weeks, depending on the degree of their kidney failure.

4 PERITONEAL DIALYSIS

This chapter concentrates on peritoneal dialysis (PD), a form of dialysis that is used to treat people with kidney failure at home.

Introduction

Peritoneal dialysis (PD) is a form of dialysis used to treat people with kidney failure at home. In PD, the process of dialysis (see Chapter 3) takes place inside the patient's body, using the peritoneum (the natural lining of the abdomen) as the dialysis membrane. PD has been available in the UK since the late 1970s and is currently the most widely used form of home dialysis.

How does PD work?

PD is a continuous treatment that takes over some of the work which is normally done by the kidneys. It removes the waste products of food that we eat, and removes excess fluid from the body.

The basic principles of dialysis are the same for PD and haemodialysis. (These principles are explained in detail in Chapter 3). Briefly, dialysis uses a special liquid (called the dialysis fluid, dialysis solution or dialysate) and a membrane (called the dialysis membrane) which acts as a filter. In PD, the dialysis membrane is the patient's own peritoneum or lining of the abdomen (see below). The dialysis membrane keeps the dialysis fluid and the blood separate from each other, and is the filter that allows certain substances and water to pass through it. Dialysis fluid is drained through a tube into the abdomen and provides the 'container' into which waste products and excess water can be removed from the body.

Substances pass from the blood into the dialysis fluid (and vice versa). They do this by a process called diffusion, by which substances pass from a stronger to a weaker solution.

At the same time, ultrafiltration occurs. Excess water passes from the blood into the dialysis fluid by a process called osmosis, in which liquid in a weaker solution passes into a stronger one. In PD, the dialysis happens continuously because there is always dialysis fluid in contact with the peritoneal membrane.

PD is a home-based therapy that patients usually do themselves. It is a flexible treatment that can be carried out anywhere there is a convenient place.

Although the vast majority of patients do PD for themselves, some patients have help from a carer to do some or all of their dialysis. This is called assisted PD.

The peritoneum

In PD, the dialysis process takes place continuously inside the patient's abdomen, using a natural membrane – the peritoneum – as the dialysis membrane. It is from the peritoneum that PD (peritoneal dialysis) gets its name.

The peritoneum is a natural membrane that lines the inside of the abdominal wall and covers all the abdominal organs (the stomach, bowels, liver, etc). It resembles a balloon in appearance and texture but has lots of extremely tiny holes in it. These holes allow the peritoneum to be used as a dialysis membrane. As blood flows through the blood vessels in the peritoneum, it flows past the holes. Although the holes are extremely tiny, water and toxins can easily pass through, but blood cells are too large. In this way, the peritoneum in PD works as a 'natural filter'.

The peritoneum has two layers – one lining the inside of the abdominal wall, the other lining the abdominal organs. Between these two layers is a space. This space is called the peritoneal cavity (see Figure 4.1). Normally, the peritoneal cavity contains only about 100 ml of liquid. During PD, it is the peritoneal cavity that is used as a reservoir for the dialysis fluid. In fact, it can expand to hold a few litres of fluid.

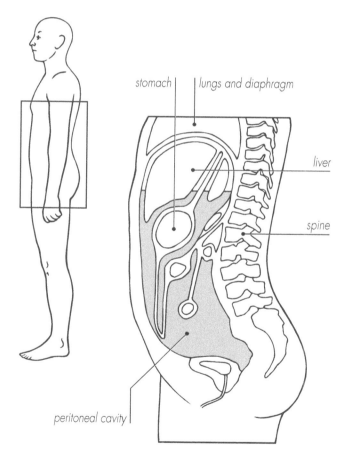

Figure 4.1: The position of the peritoneal cavity

How is PD done?

PD is a continuous therapy meaning that the levels of waste products and fluid in the body do not rise and fall as much as they do with unit-based haemodialysis (which is usually done three times a week). Dialysis takes place all the time as the fluid is constantly in contact with the peritoneal membrane. The process consists of the following three stages:

1 The peritoneal cavity is filled with between 1.5–3 litres of dialysis fluid from a dialysis bag. (The amount varies, depending on a patient's individual needs and the type of dialysis fluid used.) The fluid drains into the peritoneal cavity by gravity through a flexible tube called a "catheter".
2 The dialysis fluid is left inside the peritoneum to allow dialysis to take place. (The length of time it stays there varies, from between 2 and 8 hours, depending on individual requirements, the time of day and the type of PD.)
3 The 'used' fluid, containing the water and waste products that the kidneys would normally have passed into the urine, is drained out of the body by gravity and is thrown away, usually down the toilet.

How does the dialysis fluid get in and out of the body?

The dialysis fluid gets in and out of the peritoneal cavity via a small plastic tube that is placed into the abdomen.

The tube is inserted during a short operation (which is performed using either a local or a general anaesthetic), and will remain in place permanently, until PD is no longer required (see Figure 4.2). This tube is called a PD catheter. It is about 30 centimetres (12 inches) long and as wide as a large pencil.

The PD catheter will be placed through your lower abdominal wall, into your peritoneal cavity. Half of the catheter lies inside your abdomen, and half lies outside.

It will come out on the right or the left usually under your navel (tummy button). The PD catheter acts as a permanent pathway into your peritoneal cavity from the

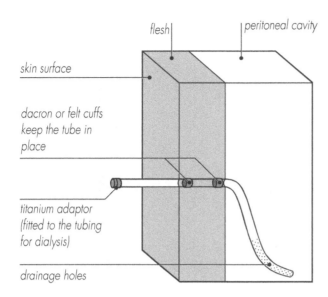

flesh

peritoneal cavity

skin surface

dacron or felt cuffs keep the tube in place

titanium adaptor (fitted to the tubing for dialysis)

drainage holes

Figure 4.2: PD catheter – position inside the body

outside world. Without it, you won't be able to perform PD, so it is important you look after it.

The operation to insert the catheter can be done as a 'day case' meaning that you won't need to stay in hospital overnight. The catheter is usually 'left alone' for 7–10 days or more after the operation. This allows it to 'settle in' and gives the abdominal wound time to heal.

Occasionally, however, it may need to be used straight away if dialysis is needed urgently.

Sometimes the PD catheter does not work first time and another short operation will be needed to resolve the problem. This might be a 'repositioning' or an 'omentectomy' (the removal of fat that has got in the way).

Learning how to do PD

PD is a home-based treatment and is usually done by patients themselves. It is important, therefore, that anyone having PD is properly trained. This training is usually given to patients, and a partner if preferred, after their

PD catheter operation and when the tube is ready to be used.

Patients are fully trained in all aspects of their care by specialist nurses. Most patients can happily do their own dialysis after about 3 to 5 days of training. Training can be done anywhere but hospitals vary. Some will train people as in-patients, meaning that you will stay in hospital to learn. Others train you as out-patients, so you will need to come into hospital each day for training. Some people are trained in their own home.

When patients first go home and have to do the dialysis by themselves, they may find it a bit daunting. However, within a few days most patients find they are doing dialysis by themselves with no problems. It is a simple process but it does need to be done carefully and meticulously.

In some situations, people are able to have support from a specially trained healthcare assistant to help with their dialysis. This is called assisted PD. This may be a temporary measure, with the healthcare assistant visiting the person for the first few weeks while confidence is built up. Other people need the support for longer, and others have permanent support.

Different types of PD

The way that the dialysis fluid is exchanged depends on the type of PD. There are two main types of PD, which differ only in the way that the dialysis fluid is exchanged.

The two different types of PD are:

1 **Continuous ambulatory peritoneal dialysis (CAPD).** 'Continuous' means 'all the time' and 'ambulatory' means 'while you walk around'. In this form of PD, the dialysis solution is changed manually.
2 **Automated peritoneal dialysis (APD).** 'Automated' means that a machine changes the dialysis fluid for the patient. The patient remains connected to the machine while dialysis is taking place, at night while they are asleep (see below).

Fluid exchanges in CAPD

CAPD involves draining between 1.5–3 litres of dialysis fluid into your abdomen, leaving it there for 4–8 hours, and then draining it out. This is done four or five times a day – every day. It is as simple as that. With practice, an exchange of fluid can be done in less than 30 minutes.

Exchanges are simple to do and can be performed almost anywhere, and you can watch TV, read or work on your laptop while it is happening.

The dialysis fluid is kept in sealed plastic bags. The bags are connected and disconnected to the peritoneal catheter with a system of tubes and clamps. (How this is done is shown in Figure 4.3).

There are no 'set' times to carry out the exchanges; however, a four-bag regime 'fits' into a typical day. For example, the first bag might be exchanged at breakfast, the second at lunchtime, the third before the evening meal, and the fourth before going to bed (leaving the fluid for the last exchange in through the night). It is easy for patients to adapt the timing of exchanges to their own individual needs. For example, if you want to go out for the day, you could delay your midday exchange, and do two 'quick bags' (say, three hours apart) after coming home. It may be safe to miss the occasional bag, but this is certainly not recommended on a regular basis. You should always check with your doctor or nurse before doing this.

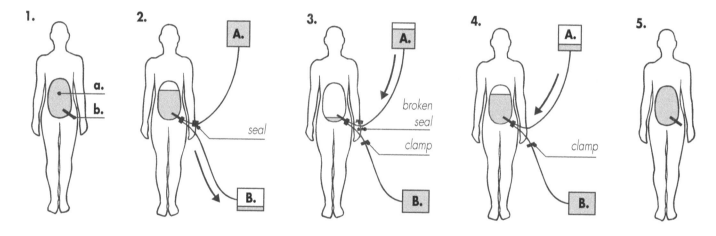

a. Peritoneal cavity
b. Catheter tube

1. Patient with used dialysis fluid ready to exchange.

2. A Y-shaped tube is connected to the patient's PD catheter. At one end of the Y tubing is a bag full of fresh dialysis fluid (A). Used fluid is drained into the empty bag (B), which is at the other end of the Y tubing.

3. When all the used fluid has drained into the drainage bag (B), the drainage tube is clamped to stop more fluid flowing down the tube. The seal is broken and fresh fluid is then drained into the peritoneal cavity from bag A.

4. Once all the fresh fluid is inside the patient, all the tubes are clamped and the bags are disconnected, leaving the patient free from the equipment until the next time a dialysis exchange is due.

5. Patient with fresh dialysis fluid.

Figure 4.3: Fluid exchanges in CAPD

Fluid exchanges in APD

APD uses a machine to do the dialysis fluid exchanges. Most people have their machine in the bedroom, where it does the exchanges while they are asleep.

APD machines are quite compact, about the size of a small suitcase (see Figure 4.4) which makes it possible for patients to do exchanges anywhere there is an electricity supply.

Most patients need to spend about 8 hours attached to the machine every night. This enables the machine to perform an average of six exchanges of dialysis fluid each night.

After spending the night on the machine, most people on APD keep fluid inside their peritoneum during the daytime without needing to exchange it until they go back onto the machine the next night.

A few patients can afford to miss one night's dialysis occasionally. However, they should always check first with the doctor or nurse at the renal unit to see whether this is safe.

The machine is programmed for each individual patient, according to their needs. The programme usually has the treatment length (how long you will stay on the machine), the fill volume (how much fluid is put into your abdomen) and if you need a different type of solution to be left inside you at the end of the treatment, which will stay there all day. This is often Icodextrin solution, which can be left in for longer than the regular glucose solution.

There is a type of APD used by some patients called 'Tidal APD'. This treatment is similar to regular APD, but the fluid isn't completely drained out at the end of each cycle. Instead, a small amount of the dialysis fluid is left inside the peritoneal cavity after each drain. New fluid is then filled and left in the abdomen as usual. This method can help some patients who have problems with their PD catheter. If the PD catheter is not positioned well inside the abdomen, it can cause some discomfort when the last little bit of fluid is drained out. Therefore, leaving a small amount at the end of each drain cycle, can prevent the discomfort.

CAPD or APD?

In most renal units in the UK, about 40% of the PD patients currently do CAPD, and 60% do APD.

Different patients may be better suited to either CAPD or APD for a number of reasons:

1 **Lifestyle choices.** APD is done during the night which means that the daytime is left free for patients to carry on their normal activities. For this reason, APD is often chosen by people who work or have a family to care for. APD is also more appropriate for people who need assistance to perform some or all of their dialysis and have assisted PD. The machine can be set up and/or dismantled by a carer, taking away some of the responsibility of dialysis.

   Some APD machines have a secure internet connection to the hospital. This means that your treatment can be monitored by the nurses and doctors looking after you. They can spot any potential problems and deal with them early, so they don't become too serious. They can also make sure that the dialysis you have been prescribed is actually what you are getting. Some systems also give the nurses and doctors the ability to change the settings on your machine remotely, through the internet. Before this feature was available the nurses would have to visit the patient at home to change the settings, or try to talk the patient through the process over the telephone.

2 **How the peritoneum works.** The main medical reason why a doctor may choose either CAPD or APD for a patient relates to the way the patient's peritoneum works during dialysis.

   Some patients have a peritoneal membrane which works best with more frequent exchanges of dialysis fluid. This type of membrane, called a 'high transport membrane' is usually more suited to APD, because the machine is able to do rapid exchanges of dialysis fluid while they sleep.

   Other patients, called 'low transporters', will get more dialysis if the fluid is left inside them for longer periods. 'Low transporters' are generally better suited to CAPD.

A test has been developed to find out whether patients are 'high' or 'low transporters'. This test is called a peritoneal equilibration test (PET) and is usually performed in hospital by a nurse. It takes place over four hours, and involves taking samples of PD fluid at 2-hourly intervals along with one blood sample. The test measures how quickly the waste products and excess water move out of the patient's bloodstream and into the dialysis fluid. If the waste products move quickly, the patient is called a 'high transporter'. If the waste products move slowly, the patient is a 'low transporter'.

3   **Patient size.** APD can also be particularly good for patients who require a lot of dialysis – for example, large people, especially those who no longer pass urine. This is because the machine can do more fluid exchanges (and therefore more dialysis), than patients are able to do themselves with CAPD. Also, as the patients are lying down, they may be more able to tolerate bigger volumes of dialysis fluid. (This is because there is less pressure on the abdomen when you are lying down.)

In these ways, APD can remove more waste products than CAPD. Even so, for some very large patients, APD during the night may not be enough. Such patients may need to do an additional CAPD exchange at tea-time.

Different amounts and types of PD fluid

Whatever the type of PD (either CAPD or APD), more toxins can be removed from the blood (i.e. clearance) by increasing either the volume of fluid used, or the number of exchanges, or both. A larger volume of dialysis fluid will remove more waste products (and a little more water) than a smaller volume of dialysis fluid.

The dialysis needs of patients depend partly on their body size (see Chapter 1). Big people usually need more fluid (2.5 or 3 litres of dialysis fluid).

The ability of PD fluid to remove water (i.e. to do ultrafiltration) is affected by the amount of glucose (sugar) in the bag – the more glucose in the bag, the more water is removed. There are three different strengths: strong (3.86% glucose solution), medium (2.27% glucose) and weak (1.36% glucose).

If you have too much water in your body (a condition called fluid overload, see Chapter 11) you will be advised to use more strong or medium dialysis fluid bags. These will remove more water than weaker dialysis fluid.

The strength of the dialysis fluid is different from the volume, or amount of dialysis fluid used in each exchange. Strong fluid has more glucose in it than a weak fluid, but the amount used will be the same.

Patients are advised to consider the weak (1.35%) fluid as their 'standard', and to try to use a minimum of stronger fluids. This is because it has been noticed that using a lot of high glucose fluid may damage the peritoneal membrane in the long term. This may mean that PD will not work effectively after many years of treatment.

Other types of dialysis solution

There are a number of other dialysis fluids available:

1   **Icodextrin.** This fluid contains a glucose polymer (in which the glucose molecules are very large), rather than ordinary glucose. Because the molecules are so large, they cannot pass through the peritoneal membrane. It is therefore good for those exchanges which take place over a longer period, either the day-time exchange for people on APD or the night-time one for people on CAPD. Icodextrin may also be recommended for PD patients who have diabetes or are overweight. This is because the glucose polymer in Icodextrin is less likely than ordinary glucose to be absorbed into the body to cause problems with sugar balance or weight gain. Icodextrin has also been shown to benefit patients who have been on PD for a

long time and whose peritoneum does not work very well for dialysis.

2 **Amino acids.** Some other dialysis fluids use amino acids (the building blocks of protein) rather than glucose. This solution does not contain any glucose, which makes it particularly suitable for people with diabetes or people who are obese.

3 **Bicarbonate.** A bicarbonate-based dialysis fluid has been developed to help patients who have problems regulating the level of acid in their bodies. The solution is very similar to that of the human body (it is 'biocompatible'), and is thought to preserve the patient's peritoneal membrane. This solution may also be good for people who experience pain when the fluid is drained in. Bicarbonate solutions are rapidly becoming the most commonly used basic solutions.

Who can have PD?

PD is suitable for most people with established renal failure (ERF). There are only two reasons why PD might not be suitable. First the patient has a serious hernia that can't be fixed with an operation. Second because the peritoneal membrane does not work. This might be due to adhesions (internal fibrous scars that form after an abdominal operation) or thickening of the peritoneal membrane. There is a condition called Encapsulating Peritoneal Sclerosis (also known as EPS) in which the peritoneal membrane can become thicker and stop working when a person has been on PD for a long time. Fortunately, this condition is extremely rare and happens to fewer than 2% of people who have been on PD for longer than eight years. If it does happen, very specialist surgeons can remove the damaged membrane during an operation. It will not be possible to have PD again following EPS.

Living with PD

PD does affect a person's lifestyle – especially because of the need for daily dialysis – but the limitations are often less of a problem than many people might expect.

1 **Flexibility.** PD is a flexible treatment which can be performed almost anywhere. The dialysis supplies can be delivered to most parts of the world, and APD machines are portable.

2 **Independence.** People on PD usually do their own dialysis, in their own homes. This gives many PD patients a greater sense of responsibility and independence than is possible for the majority of haemodialysis patients (who receive their dialysis from nurses or dialysis technicians in a hospital).

3 **Sport and exercise.** Most types of sport and exercise are possible for people on PD. Even contact sports are possible (although not always recommended).

4 **Swimming/baths/showers.** It's possible for PD patients to go swimming. Before a swim (or bath or shower), you will need to cover your PD catheter with a special plastic dressing, which you will be able to get either from your renal clinic or from your family doctor. After a swim (or bath or shower), you will need to clean the exit site of your catheter and, if possible, also do a fluid exchange.

5 **Sex.** Most people stay sexually active while on PD. Some people may find it uncomfortable to have sex with the dialysis fluid in, but they can drain it out first and use a new bag afterwards. Patients on APD can have sex during dialysis or before or after the dialysis starts. The connecting lead for the APD machine is very long and need not restrict you.

6 **Stability.** As PD takes place continually, all day and all night, people on PD generally feel fairly well most of the time. This is because their bodies do not have to put up with the rise and fall of toxins or fluid levels in the blood experienced by people who are on haemodialysis three times a week.

Delivery and storage of supplies

PD is a home-based therapy and so requires regular delivery and storage of supplies. The bags of dialysis fluid come in boxes of two, four or five. So a month's supplies can be as many as 40 boxes. These can be stored in a cupboard under the stairs, a spare bedroom, the shed or even the garage.

Most people receive a delivery of supplies once a month, although patients with very small houses or flats may be able to arrange fortnightly deliveries. The people who deliver the supplies deliver to many other dialysis patients, and are specially recruited and trained to go into patients' homes. They will move the supplies to exactly where a patient wants them, and will even move boxes around so that fluid from previous deliveries gets used before the new stock.

Possible problems with PD

PD is not always entirely trouble-free. Patients may experience various emotional and physical problems:

Emotional problems

PD requires commitment as people have to do dialysis every day. Some patients do not like the way PD affects their appearance. The abdomen may appear slightly rounded. Keeping fit and doing exercises to strengthen the abdominal muscles will help.

The PD catheter can also cause body image problems. Some people find this very difficult to cope with and may worry that it might put off a sexual partner. (See Chapter 9 for more information about the psychological aspects of kidney failure.)

Physical problems

1 **Fluid overload.** PD can remove the build-up of excess fluid that healthy kidneys would usually remove. However, in some people, either PD doesn't remove enough fluid or the person has taken too much fluid in, meaning that they will have fluid overload. This can cause swelling of the ankles and breathlessness. Fluid overload can be improved by using stronger dialysis fluid and by drinking less.

2 **Backache.** Some PD patients find that the dialysis fluid in their abdomen is uncomfortable and can cause backache.

3 **Poor drainage.** This can have a number of causes. The PD catheter may become blocked with a substance called fibrin, which is a form of protein. This looks like tiny strands of cotton wool and is completely harmless. It is easily cleared by squeezing the tubing. Alternatively, a nurse will be able to clear the catheter by injecting a de-clotting agent, called heparin, down the catheter. This is a simple procedure and will not need an operation.

   Another common reason for poor drainage is constipation. This can cause the bowels to press against the catheter and make the dialysis fluid drain very slowly. So it is very important to avoid constipation, perhaps by taking regular laxatives.

4 **Leaks.** Dialysis fluid can leak from around the tube if the catheter has not been given time to heal before it is used. If a leaking catheter is 'rested' (not used for dialysis) for 2–4 weeks, it will usually 'seal up' again, and become watertight.

5 **Hernias.** A hernia occurs when a wall of muscle weakens and lets an organ or tissue bulge through from inside. If an existing hernia is noticed by the surgeon during an operation to insert a PD catheter, it will be repaired during the same operation to stop it causing problems in the future. If a hernia occurs at a later date, it should also be repaired. This may require a 4–6 week period of haemodialysis while the operation heals.

6 **Infection.** All dialysis patients are prone to infections. Although they can usually be treated with antibiotics, it is better to avoid getting an infection in the first place. This can be achieved by strict attention to hygiene. Care is needed both with personal hygiene and when the dialysis is performed.

An infection of the peritoneum is called peritonitis. It is usually caused by germs getting into the dialysis fluid when the exchange is done. This can happen if a person touches the connection between the bag of fluid and the catheter. Being scrupulously clean during the exchange procedure can reduce the risk. While many people on PD never get an infection, some will get one once every couple of years, some will get one more frequently.

Occasionally, a patient may get several attacks of peritonitis in a row. The doctor may then decide that an operation to replace the PD catheter is needed.

Another type of infection, called an exit site infection, may also occur. This causes a red tender area around the exit site (the point where the PD catheter comes out through the skin). Keeping the catheter taped down to the skin will help reduce the risk of an exit site infection.

Keeping the exit site clean and dry will also help reduce the risk of an infection. Many people will also use an antibiotic cream. The cream is put into each nostril, which is where many of the germs that cause exit site infections live. This has been proven to significantly reduce the risk of infection.

Exit site infections respond well to antibiotics, usually given as tablets or creams.

Occasionally, an exit site infection spreads down the catheter 'tunnel' (the route taken by the catheter through the abdominal wall). If antibiotics are not effective, an operation to remove the catheter will be necessary. It is usually possible to insert a new catheter at the same operation.

KEY FACTS

1 In peritoneal dialysis (PD), the process of dialysis takes place inside the patient's abdomen.

2 PD is suitable for most people with ERF.

3 Your own peritoneum (abdominal lining) acts as the dialysis membrane.

4 There are two types of PD: CAPD (a manual technique that you do) and APD (an automated technique that a machine does). In the UK, 40% of patients have CAPD, and 60% have APD.

5 Dialysis fluid is drained into the peritoneal cavity, left there until dialysis has taken place, and is then drained out.

6 You will be trained to do the dialysis yourself, in your own home.

7 One advantage of PD is the independence it gives you. It enables you to take control of your own life and look after yourself at home.

8 You will need storage space in your home to accommodate supplies of dialysis fluid.

9 Problems with PD include infections and hernias, although many patients never experience any problems.

5 HAEMODIALYSIS

This chapter describes haemodialysis (often known as HD), which is a form of dialysis used to treat people with established kidney failure. It can be done in a hospital, a satellite unit, or at home.

Introduction

Haemodialysis treatment became routinely available in the 1960s. Although the basic principles of haemodialysis haven't changed since then, the way that the treatment happens has been developed over the years.

People who go to the hospital renal unit or a satellite unit have their dialysis on average three times a week for about four hours each time. Home-based haemodialysis, however, is usually done more frequently – up to six times a week for just a few hours a day or fewer times a week, overnight while the person is sleeping.

Currently, out of all the people who are having haemodialysis in the UK, about 5% are having their HD at home. This means that 95% of patients have their treatment in the hospital or at a 'satellite' dialysis unit which may be at local hospital or other clinic. These days, Home HD is becoming much more popular and there is some evidence to show that when HD is done more often, patients feel better, need to take fewer medicines and have a better quality of life.

How does haemodialysis work?

For dialysis to work, the dialysis fluid needs to come into contact with the patient's blood. In haemodialysis, large amounts of blood need to be removed from the body to be put through the filter. This is done through a fistula, graft or neck line.

Haemodialysis access (HD fistulas, grafts and neck lines)

In haemodialysis (or HD), 'access' is the word used to describe how access is made to the bloodstream so that dialysis can take place.

During HD, large quantities of blood must be rapidly removed from the body, and (at the same time) just as rapidly returned to it. Therefore, in most cases, HD access has two 'sides'. One of these (called the 'arterial side') is used to take blood out of the patient's body. The other (called the 'venous side') is used to return blood to the patient after dialysis.

There are three main types of access:
- A fistula, which is made from the patient's own blood vessels by joining a vein to an artery (see Figure 5.1);
- A 'graft' where a small piece of artificial tubing is used to join a vein to an artery; and
- A dialysis 'venous' catheter, which is usually a double-barrelled plastic tube (see Figure 5.2).

Fistulas

The most used form of access for haemodialysis is the arteriovenous fistula or AVF (often simply called a fistula).

Fistulas are usually preferable to catheters because they do not use any plastic, and so are less likely to become infected. A fistula will generally last longer than a catheter and often give a better dialysis quality.

Fistulas are made by a surgeon in a small operation, which may be performed under a general anaesthetic (when you are put to sleep) or a local anaesthetic (where you stay awake). In this operation, a vein (a blood vessel that carries blood back to the heart) is joined to an artery (a blood vessel that carries blood away from the heart) (see Figure 5.1). This can be done under the skin, usually at either the wrist or the elbow.

The blood pressure in arteries is always higher than the blood pressure in veins. When a fistula is formed, blood from the artery flows into the vein, and causes it to enlarge a little and the wall of the vein to thicken a bit. Once the fistula has 'matured' (i.e. grown big and strong) it will be ready for dialysis. This usually takes about six weeks. If a patient is approaching the need for haemodialysis reasonably slowly, it will be possible to plan ahead and create the fistula at the best time. There will be a best time.

1. *Normal vein.*

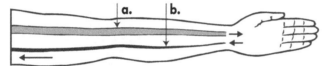

a. *Artery takes blood to the arm and hand.*
b. *Vein takes blood from the hand and arm.*

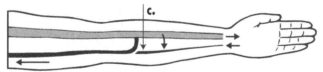

c. *A diversion of the vein is formed, linking it to the artery in the forearm.*

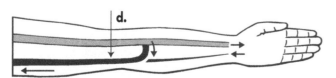

d. *The vein thickens beyond the link, and can now be used as a fistula.*

Figure 5.1: A fistula

If the fistula is made too early, it will have to wait to be used which is not ideal. But if it is too late, it will not be ready in time when the patient really does need dialysis. Most doctors would advise creating the fistula about six months before dialysis becomes necessary and gives time for the operation to be repeated if it is unsuccessful first time.

Fistulas do not always work very well and sometimes they do not work at all. It's a good idea to talk to the person that will be making your fistula (usually the surgeon) to help you to understand more about the operation and their experience.

Grafts

An 'arteriovenous' graft uses a small length of tubing (normally made of Gore-Tex®) to join an artery to a vein. The operation is done in a very similar way to a fistula under general anaesthetic by a surgeon. It is the least commonly used type of access and in most cases is used when a fistula is no longer possible.

A graft may be used sooner than a fistula because it does not need as much time to 'mature'. However, forward planning is always good. The needles are inserted through the skin into the graft tubing, whereas when a fistula is used the needles placed through the skin directly into the vein itself.

Compared to a fistula, a graft offers the same quality of dialysis but tends to last less time. It also has a higher risk of getting infected. Just like a fistula, a graft may not always work so well and will sometimes fail completely.

Catheters

A haemodialysis catheter is a plastic tube, usually with two separate barrels, one for removing blood from the body, and the other for returning it when it has passed through the dialysis filter (the dialyser). The catheter, which needs to be half in and half out of the body, is inserted during a short operation. This operation may be performed under either a general or a local anaesthetic.

The catheter is inserted into a large vein either at the

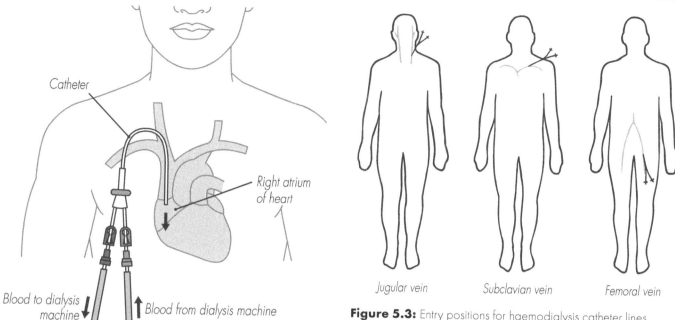

Figure 5.2: Dialysis 'venous' catheter in situ

Figure 5.3: Entry positions for haemodialysis catheter lines

side of the neck, under the collar bone, or at the top of the leg next to the groin (see Figure 5.3). Names sometimes used for catheters in these different places are a 'jugular line' (at the side of the neck), a 'subclavian line' (under the collar bone), and a 'femoral line' (in the groin). It can be used for haemodialysis almost immediately after it is inserted.

Dialysis catheters may be temporary or semi-permanent.

Temporary catheters are often used while patients are waiting for a fistula to be created. Other patients – particularly those with diabetes – have blood vessels that are not strong enough for a fistula, and will need a semi-permanent catheter for haemodialysis access.

Semi-permanent catheters are tunnelled deeper under the skin than temporary catheters. They also have small cuffs around them, just under the skin, to help keep them in place, and to help keep germs out

of the body. Semi-permanent catheters also tend to be softer and more flexible than most temporary catheters. These are often used when a patient's fistula has stopped working.

After each dialysis session, saline (salt dissolved in water) is injected into the line to remove any blood. The inside of the catheter may then be filled with a drug called heparin. Heparin stops the formation of blood clots, which could block the catheter. This keeps the catheter clear of clots between dialysis sessions. In some hospitals, the dialysis catheter is injected with antibiotics after use to prevent infections.

Between dialysis sessions, patients are asked to keep their catheter clean and dry, and to ensure that it has a dressing on it at all times.

Without access, patients who are treated by haemodialysis cannot dialyse. It is therefore very important that everyone – doctors, nurses and patients – all treat catheters and fistulas with great care.

What happens during HD?

During haemodialysis, blood is taken from the body and pumped around a dialysis machine and through a dialyser. In the dialyser, waste products and excess water pass from the blood into the dialysis fluid. The cleansed blood is then returned to the body at the same rate at which it is removed. Meanwhile, the 'used' dialysis fluid (full of waste products and extra water) is pumped out of the dialysis machine and down the drain.

Haemodialysis is a treatment that takes over some of the work normally done by the kidneys. It removes the waste products of food and removes excess water from the body.

The basic principles of dialysis are explained in detail in Chapter 3. Briefly, dialysis uses a special liquid (called the dialysis fluid, dialysis solution or dialysate) and a membrane (called the dialysis membrane) to do some of the work of the kidneys.

In haemodialysis, the process of dialysis occurs in an artificial filter through a machine. This machine is called a dialysis machine or kidney machine (see Figure 5.4). Blood from the patient is pumped through the machine so that dialysis can take place.

The filter, called the dialyser or artificial kidney (see Figure 5.5) is a cylinder that contains thousands of very small hollow tubes. Each of the tubes is made from very thin plastic, which acts as the dialysis membrane. The patient's blood is pumped through the middle of the tubes. Meanwhile, the machine pumps dialysis fluid around the outside of the tubes. The process of dialysis takes place through microscopic holes in the tubes. Various substances and water can easily pass through the holes, but blood cells cannot.

During dialysis, wastes (such as creatinine and urea) pass from the blood into the dialysis fluid. They do this by a process called diffusion, by which substances pass from a stronger to a weaker solution.

Haemodialysis also balances some of the other substances that are needed by the body. This also happens during the diffusion process. Some substances such as

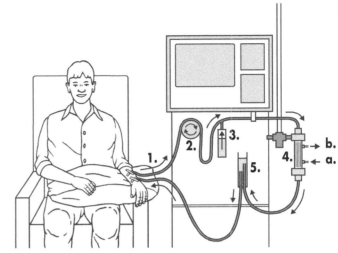

1. *Blood comes from the arm.*
2. *Blood is pumped through the machine.*
3. *Heparin (a drug to prevent clotting) is added to the blood.*
4. *Blood enters the dialyser. Dialysis fluid with treated water (a) enters the dialyser, and wastes are taken away to a drain (b).*
5. *Blood passes through a bubble trap.*
6. *Blood goes back to the arm.*

Figure 5.4: How a dialysis machine works

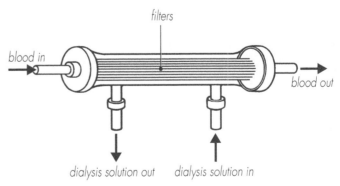

Figure 5.5: A dialyser (artificial kidney)

sodium (salt), potassium and calcium can be removed from the blood during dialysis by diffusion. However, if the body is short of some of these other substances (such as bicarbonate) they can be put into the body from the dialysis fluid. Again, it is diffusion (now working in the opposite direction) that makes this possible.

The second main function of the kidneys (and therefore of dialysis) is to remove water. In haemodialysis, it is the action of the dialysis machine that removes the water. The machine applies a sucking pressure, or negative pressure that draws water out of the blood and into the dialysis fluid. This process is known as ultrafiltration or 'u...f...ing'.

Instructions about the amount of water to be removed and the rate of ultrafiltration are entered into the machine at the start of each dialysis session, depending on how much excess water the patient has to lose.

The quality (or efficiency) of HD can be affected by a number of different things:

- How long (how many hours) and how often (how many days a week) the dialysis is done.
- The length of the gap between dialysis sessions. There is some research that shows having more than one day off between dialysis treatments can be very harmful.
- How quickly and how much blood flows through the dialyser during the treatment. This depends on how well the patient's dialysis access (their fistula, graft or catheter) is working.
- The speed at which the dialysis fluid flows on the opposite side of the dialysis membrane to the blood.
- The size of the holes in the dialysis membrane (the dialyser) and the size of the membrane surface area inside the dialyser.
- The temperature of the dialysis fluid. It is thought that cooler dialysis fluid can give a better quality of dialysis.

What is haemodiafiltration (HDF) and how does it work?

Haemodialysis (HD), described in the section above, uses the process of diffusion to remove (or replace) most of the substances that are not in balance in the body. However, haemodialysis isn't very good at getting rid of some of the slightly bigger substances from the blood. This is the case even if a dialyser is used which has slightly bigger holes. These substances are called 'middle molecules' and build-up of them is thought to be harmful to dialysis patients.

However, these middle molecules can be removed during dialysis using a slightly different process which is called 'convection'. Haemodiafiltration (HDF) is a dialysis method that uses two principles – diffusion and convection. Convection moves large amounts water across the membrane. This process is done by taking much more water out of the patient's blood through the dialyser (filter) so that the middle molecules are removed along with the water. It's almost like flushing the extra substances out of the blood.

Taking too much water from the patient's blood during dialysis could be harmful, so some water is put back into the blood as soon as it comes out of the dialyser. This technique is called 'Post Dilution HDF'.

There is another type of HDF called 'Pre Dilution HDF' which is when water is put into the blood before it goes through the dialyser. Then, high volumes of water can be removed from the blood while it flows through the dialyser, taking the middle molecules with it.

This extra water is made from the dialysis fluid which is made by the dialysis machine; it is called 'on-line' fluid.

Doctors think that post-dilution HDF is better than pre-dilution HDF because it removes more of the middle molecules and other substances.

HDF works best when the blood flows through the dialyser quickly. A rate of more than 350 mls every minute is thought to be best. Not every patient has a fistula (or graft or catheter) that can take more than 350 mls of blood a minute from their body, so HDF isn't always beneficial for everyone.

Some newer dialyses (filters) can remove middle molecules without the need for HDF.

What is High Dose HD and how does it work?

High Dose HD is HD (or HDF) which is done more often than three times a week for four hours. Most of the people who have dialysis in a satellite unit or the main renal unit will have their dialysis three times a week – either on a Monday, Wednesday and Friday or on Tuesday, Thursday and Saturday. This means that every week all these patients will have two days together off dialysis, either on a Saturday and Sunday or on a Sunday and Monday.

Some research was done in 2015 to look at the effect that taking two consecutive days off dialysis has on patients. This and other research showed that taking two days off dialysis together can be bad for patients' health. During these two days, excess fluid and wastes build up in the body more than they do when there is only a day between dialysis. This can put extra strain on the heart. Also, when HD is done three times a week, patients can take a long time to recover after each dialysis session.

Having dialysis more often, either for 2–3 hours every day, on alternate days for four hours or overnight while sleeping, for 5 or 6 days a week, has shown to have very many health benefits. In conclusion, this study showed that (compared to the normal way of doing dialysis three times a week) more frequent haemodialysis improved the health of the heart and reduced the need for patients to take blood pressure medications. It also improved some of the bone problems patients have, and improved some aspects of patients' quality of life.

High Dose HD can be done in the hospital or satellite unit but it is much easier to organise for people who have their dialysis at home, as they can be more flexible with the times that they do their treatment.

Getting involved in your dialysis and sharing care

Some kidney doctors and nurses encourage their patients to become more involved in their dialysis. This has many advantages for patients as it has been shown that people who are more involved with their own care, and who do more for themselves, can have a better quality of life and have fewer symptoms.

Over many years, it has been common practice for patients to be dialysed by the staff in haemodialysis centres unless they choose to train to dialyse at home. In recent years, some haemodialysis centres or units have involved patients in their own care and treatment in the dialysis unit. One such example from the UK, the Shared Haemodialysis Care programme, set up in 2010, gives patients the opportunity to be more independent in-centre by offering support and education to be more involved and undertake a range of tasks for themselves.

Much like patients who do their dialysis at home, this has many advantages for patients. It has been shown that people who are more involved with their care understand more about their condition, feel more in control and can have a better quality of life. Patients can get involved at any level that suits and interests them. They can learn the small tasks, such as how to take and record their blood pressure and weight, or they can learn some or all of the more complex tasks, such as setting up the dialysis machine and putting needles into their fistula.

There is a wide range of tasks that patients can become involved with. They can learn any part of any task. It's all about choice, and engaging at a level that suits the patient as an individual.

This is a typical list of tasks that patients can get involved in:

- Observations such as weight, blood pressure and temperature;
- Setting up the dialysis machine;
- Preparing the dressing pack;
- Programming the dialysis machine with personal prescription details;

- Inserting needles or preparing their neck line;
- Connecting to the dialysis machine and commencing dialysis;
- Monitoring condition and problems during dialysis;
- Discontinuing dialysis;
- Administering any medications.

This approach may help patients to become more independent. Some patients doing shared care find that they gain the confidence to consider the option of training to do their own dialysis, either at home or in the unit.

You can find out more about Shared HD on their website www.shareddialysis-care.org.uk.

Living with HD

HD will affect your lifestyle, particularly if you need to travel to a renal unit for treatment. Home HD can also have an impact as you'll need somewhere to do the dialysis and somewhere to store equipment.

1 **Flexibility.** Unit based HD is not as flexible as Home HD. If you have your dialysis in the unit, you will be given a 'slot', usually three times a week. This could be every Monday, Wednesday and Friday at say 8am to 12pm, or every Tuesday, Thursday and Saturday at say 1pm to 5pm. These are fixed but you may be able to swap your session with another patient if you have a special request.

   Home HD is more flexible and you can do the dialysis when it is convenient; after work, during the night while you sleep, or while watching television.

2 **Time.** Each HD session in the renal unit usually lasts for about four hours (some people may spend more or less time on the machine, depending on individual needs). However, travelling to and from the unit also takes time and will depend on how far you live from the unit, and what form of transport you use. Transport provided by the hospital can take a while, and there are sometimes delays. This can be because a number of patients all travel together to and from the dialysis unit.

If one patient is delayed, the others will need to wait before the transport can leave. Traffic can also cause delays!

3 **Independence.** You can be as involved in your dialysis as you choose. Those people who have Home HD will be trained to do their own treatment, along with a partner if they wish. Shared Care in a renal unit is a great way to start becoming more independent.

4 **Sport and exercise.** Most types of sport and exercise are possible for people on HD. Even contact sports are possible (although not always recommended) and it is really important to protect your fistula to prevent damage.

5 **Swimming/baths/showers.** It is possible for HD patients to go swimming; however, it is not recommended if you have a temporary dialysis catheter. For people who have dialysis catheters, waterproof dressings are provided which should be used when bathing.

6 **Sex.** Most people stay sexually active while on dialysis, although many people with kidney failure suffer from tiredness which may cause problems.

7 **Stability.** Unlike PD, HD is not a continuous treatment and so the levels of waste and extra water can build up in the body in between treatments. This can make people feel 'washed-out' after a dialysis treatment, or unwell when they have had the long break between sessions. Having HD more frequently, which can be done with Home HD, will prevent this water and waste build up and so remove this potential problem.

Having HD at home

Setting up your home for HD will require some planning and alterations to your house. The HD machine will need to be installed along with a special water treatment machine. When deciding where to put the dialysis machine you need to consider:

- **Where will you have your dialysis?** Think about the time of day you will be doing your treatment and therefore what the best place in the house would be. For example, if you decide to have Home HD overnight, the machine can be put in the bedroom. If you prefer to have Home HD during the daytime, you could have the machine placed in a spare room or a living room.

- **Space**. It is important to have enough space around the machine to allow easy access for setting up and cleaning. It is advisable to have at least one square metre.
- **Water supply.** There needs to be a water supply to the machine and this usually requires a water pressure of at least 1.5 bar. The hospital technicians can check this for you.
- **Waste plumbing.** As well as a water supply, there also needs to be a waste pipe installed to enable the waste dialysis fluid to be sent down the drain.
- **Electricity supply.**

Having Home HD requires regular delivery and storage of supplies. The dialysis supplies will include dialysis solutions, needles, tubing for the dialysis machine and equipment for cleaning and dressings. Most people have a delivery every couple of months but this can be more frequent if you don't have a lot of storage space. The equipment can be stored in a cupboard under the stairs, a spare bedroom, the shed or even the garage.

The people who deliver the supplies deliver to many other dialysis patients, and are specially recruited and trained to go into patients' homes. They will move the supplies to exactly where a patient wants them, and will even move boxes around so that stock from previous deliveries gets used before the new stock.

Possible problems with HD

Life on any form of dialysis isn't always easy and HD patients may experience various emotional and physical problems.

Emotional problems

Any form of dialysis requires commitment as people have to do dialysis frequently. Going to the hospital on a regular basis can make some people feel depressed and a 'burden' to those close to them. It can be a worry if the dialysis schedule affects your work. Many employers do understand and can accommodate the changes required. The doctors and nurses in the hospital can help talk to your employer if needed.

Some patients do not like the way the fistula looks and so always wear long sleeves to cover their arms. Also, some people find it difficult to tell friends or family about their dialysis. See Chapter 9 for more details about emotional problems and how to cope.

Physical problems

1   **Fluid overload.** HD removes the build-up of excess fluid that healthy kidneys would usually remove. However, if the person has taken too much fluid in between dialysis treatments, they will have fluid overload. This can cause swelling of the ankles and breathlessness. Fluid overload can be improved by having dialysis and by drinking less.
2   **Low blood pressure (hypotension).** This is one of the most common problems for people who use HD. It is most often caused because the body's fluid levels drop quickly during the dialysis session. This is more likely to happen if the patient needs to remove a lot of fluid because they are fluid overloaded. Low blood pressure can make you feel sick and dizzy. Low blood pressure can be avoided by keeping to your daily fluid allowance.
3   **Muscle cramps.** Some people suffer from cramps, particularly in their legs, during HD. Cramp can be caused by the body's reaction to having a lot of fluid removed in a short period of time.
4   **Problems with blood access.** HD relies on the machine being able to filter a large amount of blood. This means that between 250 and 400 mls (about ¾ pint) of blood is taken from the body via the fistula

(or venous catheter) every minute during a dialysis session. If the fistula or catheter doesn't work properly, this causes problems with the dialysis and can make it less effective.

5 **Infections**. All dialysis patients are prone to infections. Although they can usually be treated with antibiotics, it is better to avoid getting an infection in the first place. This can be achieved by strict attention to hygiene. Care is needed both with personal hygiene and when the dialysis is performed.

HD takes blood out of the body during each dialysis session for it to be filtered. There is a risk that the blood can become infected during the dialysis if care isn't taken. An infection of the blood is called 'sepsis' and can be life threatening. The fistula itself may also become infected if it isn't cleaned properly before and after treatment.

Another type of infection, called an exit site infection, may also occur. This causes a red tender area around the exit site (the point where the venous catheter comes out through the skin). Keeping the catheter covered with a dressing and taped down to the skin will help reduce the risk of an exit site infection.

KEY FACTS

1 In haemodialysis (HD), the process of dialysis takes place outside the patient's body by passing their blood through a filter.

2 Haemodialysis can be done at home or in a hospital renal unit.

3 HD in a renal unit is usually done for about 4 hours three times a week. Patients need to travel to and from the renal unit to have their treatment, which can make the process longer.

4 HD can be done more frequently than three times a week and has many advantages, including taking fewer medicines and often feeling a lot better.

5 People who chose Home HD will be trained to do the dialysis themselves but the nurses from the hospital are there to support.

6 You will need storage space in your home to accommodate supplies of dialysis fluid.

7 Problems with HD include infections and cramps, although some patients don't experience problems.

6 TRANSPLANTATION

This chapter provides information about kidney transplants. It covers the issues and the various actions that are necessary before a patient can have the operation, what happens during the operation and what you can expect afterwards.

Introduction

A kidney transplant involves removing a healthy kidney from one person (the donor) and giving it to another person (the recipient). Transplant kidneys may come from a person who has given a kidney after their death or from a living donor. Living donor kidneys may come from people who are related to the recipient or who are unrelated to the recipient.

Who can have a transplant?

About 30% of patients with kidney failure are suitable for a transplant provided the right donor kidney can be found. Anyone with serious heart or lung disease, or who has been diagnosed with cancer may not be suitable for a kidney transplant.

There isn't really an age limit for receiving a kidney transplant. In fact about 30% of kidney transplants in the UK are given to people over the age of 65. However, most renal units would think very seriously before transplanting a patient who is over 80 years old. As with many medical treatments the risk of side effects and complications does go up as we get older so balancing the risk and benefit of transplantation is very important.

Why is a kidney transplant the best option for people who can have one?

A successful kidney transplant is the most effective treatment for kidney failure compared to either peritoneal dialysis or haemodialysis. This is because a well-functioning transplanted kidney can do all the jobs of the kidney, whereas dialysis only really replaces a couple of functions. A 'good' transplant provides about 60% of the function of two normal kidneys, compared with only about 5–10% from either type of dialysis. So, a stable transplant patient with a well-functioning kidney will still have chronic kidney failure at Stage 2 or 3.

A kidney transplant can also improve quality of life. The most obvious advantage of a transplant to people with kidney failure is freedom from dialysis. There are also no particular fluid or dietary restrictions after a transplant. Erythropoietin and phosphate binder tablets can usually be stopped. Most people who have had a transplant feel better and have more energy than they did on dialysis. Women are more likely to get pregnant and have a healthy baby.

There is no doubt that for the right patient at the right time, a transplant is the best treatment option. However, not all patients are suitable for a transplant, and not all suitable patients are suitable all the time.

To enable a transplant to work properly, it is vital that patients take medicines to stop their body from rejecting the transplanted kidney. These medicines need to be taken every single day.

What are the risks?

Although a transplant is an excellent treatment for most people with ERF, it is not problem-free. Some people who have had a transplant experience a problem called rejection. This is the main reason why transplants do not last for ever.

In addition to rejection, other problems that a patient may experience after a transplant include:

- drug side effects;
- infection;
- heart disease;
- cancer;
- the return of the disease that originally caused the kidneys to fail.

Rejection

Rejection is a condition when the patient's body recognises that the transplanted kidney is not 'its own' and tries to 'reject' it from the body. Even when patients and transplant kidneys are apparently 'well matched' in terms of blood group and tissue type, some degree of rejection is common.

Rejection may be either acute or chronic.

The body's immune system is responsible for the rejection process. The immune system is the body's natural defence system. It has many different parts and includes organs such as the spleen and appendix, the lymph nodes and specialist white blood cells (called lymphocytes).

The usual task of the immune system is to fight foreign invaders. These include germs and foreign objects (such as splinters or thorns embedded in the skin). The immune system also fights cancer.

A person's immune system does not usually attack its own body because the cells have a 'friendly face' ('self-antigens' on the outer surface of the cells). These cells are taken out of action by the immune system.

The immune system is important because it protects the body from dangerous infections, foreign bodies and cancer. However, after a transplant it can be a problem.

If the immune system recognises that the new kidney does not have the usual friendly face of the body's own cells, it will become overactive and send lymphocytes to attack and reject the kidney. The body is actually trying to protect you from the kidney, which it perceives as a danger.

To prevent this from happening there are drugs – called immunosuppressant drugs – that dampen down the immune system to prevent or treat the rejection process, while still keeping it active enough to fight infection. Finding the balance can be difficult.

All patients who have a kidney transplant need to take immunosuppressant drugs.

Most transplant patients will take two or three different kinds of immunosuppressant drugs every day. If they stop taking these drugs, the immune system 'fights back' and the kidney will be rejected by the body and stop working.

Because of the constant threat of rejection, it is very important never to run out of immunosuppressant drugs. If you do run out it is important to go to the hospital at once. If you have diarrhoea and vomiting, it can prevent the drugs from being absorbed by your body and so they won't work properly. The immune system never forgets that there is a 'foreign' kidney in the body. It is always waiting for a chance to attack and reject it. That's why taking the medicines every day is so important.

Many other medicines can interact with immunosuppressant drugs. So patients should always check with the kidney unit pharmacist, or hospital doctor, before taking any new medication.

Acute rejection. 'Acute' means short term, coming on quickly and needing immediate action. Acute rejection can happen in the first few months (particularly the first few weeks) after a transplant. It is very common – about 40% of patients experience acute rejection in the first year after a transplant. If acute rejection hasn't happened within one year of the operation, then it is unlikely to happen, unless the patient stops taking their drugs correctly.

Stopping immunosuppressant drugs can cause acute rejection at any time.

Acute rejection may sometimes cause pain and fever, but usually there are no symptoms. Doctors will suspect that a patient has acute rejection if the blood creatinine level is high after the transplant.

Before rejection can be diagnosed, a number of tests are done to make sure that the blood supply to the kidney is still working and there are no other blockages or problems.

The only way to be sure whether a transplant kidney is being rejected is to do a kidney biopsy. This is when a very tiny piece of the kidney is taken out so that it can be examined under a microscope.

If the biopsy shows signs of rejection, the patient will usually be given rejection therapy drugs (see below).

Chronic rejection. 'Chronic' means long term and of slow onset. It is very different from acute rejection. In chronic rejection, there is no real rejection process taking place. The patient's immune system does not attack and reject the transplant kidney in the same way as it does in acute rejection. This is why it is sometimes called 'transplant glomerulopathy' rather than 'rejection'.

Chronic rejection is more like a slow ageing of the new kidney. If it happens, it will usually be more than a year after the transplant operation.

As with acute rejection the only sure way to diagnose the condition is to do a biopsy. There is no treatment for chronic rejection.

The severity of chronic rejection varies. Mild chronic rejection is not usually a problem. However, more severe chronic rejection will eventually lead to failure of the kidney. If this happens the patient will need to go back onto dialysis or have another transplant.

Medicines for kidney transplants
Immunosuppressant drugs
There is no immunosuppressant drug that has been proven to be better than all the rest. Their effectiveness depends on each patient, how they respond to each drug and their medical conditions. Many drugs are now available. If a patient has side effects from a particular drug, it can be changed for an alternative. The choice of drugs is influenced partly by the cost.

Induction therapy. Induction therapy is the name given to the drugs that are used for patients at the time of the kidney transplant operation to prevent acute kidney transplant rejection in the early days. The drugs basiliximabor daclizumab are most commonly used for this.

Maintenance therapy. This is the name given to the drugs that are taken long term to prevent rejection. The most widely used drugs for maintenance therapy are tacrolimus and mycophenolate. Some patients may also need to take a low dose of a steroid such as prednisolone. Maintenance therapy is taken for as long as the transplant kidney continues to work.

Sometimes, other drugs are given to patients for maintenance therapy. This may be because the side effects of tacrolimus and mycophenolate are too harmful, or it might be because they need to be given in such high doses that the drugs actually harm the transplant kidney. See below for more details on the side effects of immunosuppression.

Rejection therapy. If a person's body does reject the transplant kidney, there are other drugs that can be taken to rescue the situation.

The patient will usually be given a high dose of a steroid drug (either prednisolone or methylprednisolone) for three days. This short-course, high-dose treatment will usually defeat the rejection process, and the blood creatinine will start to decrease. If the steroids do not work, the immunosuppressant tablets may be changed to a slightly 'stronger' drug.

Alternatively, the patient may be given a 5–10 day course of a stronger intravenous injection, such as antilymphocyte globulin (ALG), anti-thymocyte globulin (ATG) or orthoclone K T-cell receptor 3 (OKT3) antibody.

These treatments almost always work, and the rejection process goes away. However, all of them can have fairly severe side effects, especially OKT3, which can cause fever, diarrhoea, joint and muscle pain, wheezing, and shortness of breath due to fluid on the lungs (pulmonary oedema).

In some patients, a treatment called plasmapheresis may be used along with these drugs. This treatment is similar to haemodialysis. A machine is used to filter the blood in a similar way. A number of plasmapheresis treatments may be required for a few weeks until the kidney starts to work again.

Drug side effects

All immunosuppressant drugs have side effects:

1 **Basiliximab and Daclizumab.** The most common side effect that these drugs cause is tummy upsets such as abdominal pain, nausea and vomiting.

2 **Tacrolimus.** If patients are given too much ciclosporin, it can be toxic (poisonous) to the kidney. This can prevent the transplant from working.

    Tacrolimus can cause hair loss. It may also lead to the patient developing diabetes which may need to be treated with insulin injections twice a day for the rest of their life. Tacrolimus can also damage the nervous system which may cause trembling.

3 **Mycophenolate.** This drug can cause abdominal pain and diarrhoea. It is also known to stop the bone marrow from working properly. The bone marrow is where blood cells are made. By affecting blood cell production, this drug can cause a number of serious problems. If too few red blood cells are produced, the patient will suffer from anaemia, causing tiredness. If there are too few white blood cells, the patient will develop a condition called neutropenia. This will affect the patient's ability to fight infection. If too few of the blood cells called platelets are produced, this can make the patient bleed or bruise easily.

4 **Ciclosporin.** If patients are given too much ciclosporin, it can be toxic (poisonous) to the kidney. This can prevent the transplant from working.

    Some patients who take ciclosporin for a long time can get gum hypertrophy. This is when the gums grow too much, which can look bad. It is less likely to develop if patients regularly floss between the teeth. It the problem becomes severe, the gums can be 'cut back' using a specialist hospital-based dental treatment.

    Another possible side effect of ciclosporin is excessive growth of hair on the face and body. It can also cause diabetes and may lead to a lifelong need for insulin injections twice a day.

    Ciclosporin can also damage the liver and nervous system.

5 **Sirolimus.** This drug is not so poisonous to the kidney. However, it can cause a very high cholesterol level in the blood. It also can slow down or prevent the healing of wounds which can cause problems after surgical operations. In addition, Sirolimus can cause tummy upsets, mouth ulcers and bone marrow suppression.

6 **Azathioprine.** This drug can also suppress activity in the bone marrow which can cause the problems described above. Patients who take Azathioprine may also get skin rashes and it can also cause damage to the liver.

    Stopping these drug or reducing the dose will normally put matters right. This should only be done on advice from your doctor.

7 **Prednisolone.** This drug is a steroid, and it can cause thinning of the skin (leading to easy bruising) and facial swelling. These problems may lessen if the dose of the drug is reduced. Prednisolone can also cause diabetes. A further possible problem with prednisolone is that it can cause damage to the joints, especially the hip joints. Pain in either hip, even in the first 3–6 months after a transplant, should be taken seriously. Using steroids for a long time can cause osteoporosis. This can cause serious damage to the spine which can be very painful, as well as reducing your height.

If they are given, the steroid tablets will probably be stopped after the first 6–12 months because of these side effects.

Getting the balance right

It is absolutely vital for the health of your kidney transplant that the right amount of anti-rejection drugs are given at the right time. To help the doctors to decide how much of each drug to give, the level of the drugs in your blood is measured. These blood tests are just as important as remembering to take your medicines every day. If the levels are either too high or too low, there is a serious risk that the transplanted kidney will stop working.

It is also important to follow the instructions from the doctors and nurses on the days when you are having your blood tests. You may be asked not to take your medicines until after the blood tests. This is so that the amount of the drug left in your bloodstream can be measured accurately. If you have the blood test just after you have taken your medicine, it may lead to a false high reading. The doctors may then (incorrectly) reduce the dose of your medicines.

If you are struggling to take your medicines, either because you forget or because you are having side effects, speak to one of the doctors or nurses at the hospital. You can even talk to your GP who will be able to offer some advice, counselling and support.

Infection

Although immunosuppressant drugs make the immune system less effective, they do not stop patients from fighting infections. So people taking immunosuppressant drugs do not necessarily get lots of infections.

However, there is one infection that is a particular problem after transplantation. It is called cytomegalovirus (CMV) infection. For most people who are not taking immunosuppressant drugs, CMV is a mild infection that causes a 'flu-like illness. However, in patients who have just received a transplant, CMV infection can be quite a severe illness.

If a transplant patient does ever get CMV, there is an effective treatment for it either as tablets or a drip. Some people who are at particular risk of getting CMV will be given tablets to prevent possible infection.

The most common infection that people experience after a kidney transplant is a urine infection. Patients therefore need to be especially aware of the symptoms of urine infections so that they can alert the doctor if they think they have one. The most common symptoms are:

- cloudy or bloody urine;
- needing to pass water more often than usual;
- foul-smelling urine;
- pain or a burning sensation when passing water;
- feeling that you need to pass water often;
- cramps or pressure in the lower abdomen or lower back.

Heart disease

Heart attacks and problems with the circulation (such as stroke and reduced blood flow to the legs) are much more common after a transplant. This is partly because of the effects of kidney failure on the circulation before a transplant.

It may be due to other problems such as high blood pressure, a high cholesterol level in the blood, diabetes (which can start after a transplant, as it is a side effect of many immunosuppressant drugs) and increased risk of clotting ('thickening') of the blood.

The risk of these problems may be reduced if the patient does not smoke, keeps fit, and keeps their weight under control.

Diabetes

Following a kidney transplant, people are more likely to develop Type 2 diabetes. The condition is known as Post Transplant Diabetes Mellitus (PTDM) and can affect up to 20% of patients within six months of the operation. This problem is becoming more and more common and may lead to patients needing to have insulin injections two or three times a day and being on a special diet again.

Therefore it is really important to try to help prevent

diabetes. This can be done by following the healthy eating guidelines, avoiding becoming overweight and keeping active by taking regular exercise.

Cancer

One of the functions of the immune system is to fight cancer. By making the immune system less efficient to help prevent transplant rejection, immunosuppressant drugs unfortunately increase the likelihood of getting some types of cancer.

Exposure to the sun greatly increases the risk of developing skin cancer. In fact, transplant patients are 30–40 times more likely to develop skin cancer. The risk for a common type of skin cancer – called squamous cell carcinoma – is 80 times higher than people who haven't had a transplant. It is therefore very important for people who have had a transplant to use a strong 'sun block' cream.

Lymphoma

About 5% of people who have had a kidney transplant will get lymphoma. This is a more serious cancer of the bone marrow and immune system. It is a bit like leukaemia. This is about 10 times more common than in people who haven't had a transplant. It is particularly common in patients who have had stronger immunosuppressant drugs.

Lymphoma sometimes 'goes away' when the doses of immunosuppressant drugs are reduced. In more severe cases it has to be treated with high doses of chemotherapy. In some cases, the immunosuppressant drugs given for the transplant are stopped, which can lead to loss of the kidney.

Although treatment can be successful, between 30 and 50% of people who get lymphoma after a transplant die within two years of the diagnosis.

New kidneys and old diseases

Patients who are having kidney transplants sometimes worry that the original cause of their kidney failure might make the new kidney fail too, but this is very unusual.

An exception, however, is where the original kidneys failed because the patient had a condition called focal and segmental glomulerosclerosis (FSGS). This disease comes back in around 20% of patients who have had it before. Patients who have lost one kidney transplant due to recurrent FSGS have a 50% chance of losing another one.

There are a few other types of kidney disease that may also come back and affect the transplanted kidney. These include mesangiocapillary glomerulonephritis, atypical haemolytic uraemic syndrome, membranous nephropathy, IgA nephropathy, Henoch-Schönlein purpura, and lupus nephritis. However, if these conditions do recur, they do not always lead to loss of the kidney transplant.

If the condition that caused your kidney failure comes back, and causes the kidney to fail in two transplants, doctors would be unlikely to recommend that you have a third transplant.

Patients who are affected by any of these conditions should ask their doctor about the likelihood of the original disease recurring, and damaging a kidney transplant.

What happens before you have a kidney transplant?

Tests for transplant suitability

Before a patient can be put forward for a transplant, they will have to be tested for infections. These include HIV (the virus that causes AIDS), hepatitis B, hepatitis C and cytomegalovirus (CMV). It is important to test for these viruses because they may be dormant ('sleeping,' causing no symptoms) in a patient's body. After the transplant, they may be 'woken up' and cause illness. This is especially true of CMV.

If a patient has one of these viruses, it does not mean that they will not get a transplant. However, knowing that the virus is there will ensure the correct treatments are given.

Refusing to have any of these tests will mean that you are unable to have a transplant.

Other tests are also necessary before a patient can have a transplant. These include an electrocardiogram (ECG, an electric recording of the heart beat), a chest X-ray, and sometimes an echocardiogram (ECHO, a soundwave picture of the heart), a myocardial perfusion scan (MPS) (a form of nuclear medicine scan) and possibly an 'exercise test' (a test in which the patient has to walk on a moving walkway, to test their fitness, and stress the heart). Some kidney units also insist that patients who have diabetes also have a cardiac catheter test (a special X-ray picture of the heart). More detailed tests on the heart may be needed, particularly for people at higher risk of heart disease.

If results of all these tests are satisfactory, the patient can then be put on the national waiting list for a deceased donor transplant, or considered for a possible transplant from a living donor.

Being ready for a transplant

Patients waiting for a deceased donor transplant will not be given very much notice that a kidney is available for them. So they need to be prepared to go to the hospital at short notice. It may be sensible to leave your mobile phone on 24 hours a day. When patients are on the transplant waiting list, it is up to them to make themselves contactable at all times, day and night. If a patient cannot be found, the kidney will be offered to someone else. When a patient 'gets the call' they should go to the hospital right away. They should not have anything to eat or drink, in preparation for the anaesthetic.

Remember that the renal centre that looks after you for pre-dialysis care and dialysis treatment may send you to a transplant centre at a different hospital for the operation.

Tests before the operation

Patients called in to the hospital for a transplant are not guaranteed to receive it. Before the operation can go ahead, it is necessary to check that the patient is well enough to have the operation, and that they will not reject the transplant kidney.

1 **Physical examination.** The purpose of a physical examination is to check that it is safe to proceed with the operation. For example, if a patient has a heavy cold, it may considered too much of a risk for them to have an anaesthetic.

2 **The cross-match.** This is a blood test that checks the patient has no antibodies (substances that normally help the body to fight infection) that would react with the donor kidney. High levels of such antibodies in the blood mean that the new kidney is likely to be rejected as soon as it is put into the patient, even if it seems a good tissue type match.

A cross-match is done by mixing a sample of the patient's blood with blood cells from the donor. If there is no reaction, it is assumed that the patient will be less likely to reject the new kidney when it is transplanted. This is called a negative cross-match, and means that the operation can go ahead.

If the cross-match is positive (i.e. there is a reaction between the patient's blood and the donor's cells), the patient will be sent home and put back on the waiting list. This can be very disappointing, but it is much better to return to dialysis for a while than to be given a kidney that doesn't work, and which may make the recipient extremely ill.

The transplant operation

An operation to transplant a kidney requires a general anaesthetic and lasts about 2 hours.

The procedure

The surgeon makes a diagonal incision (cut) into the abdomen, on the right or the left, below the navel (see Figure 6.1).

The patient's own kidneys are usually left in place. The transplant kidney is placed lower down in the

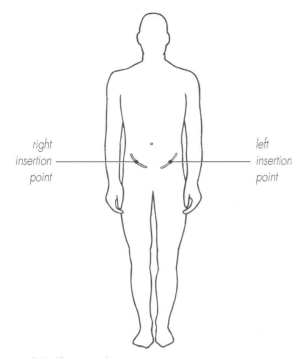

Figure 6.1: The transplant operation: incision sites

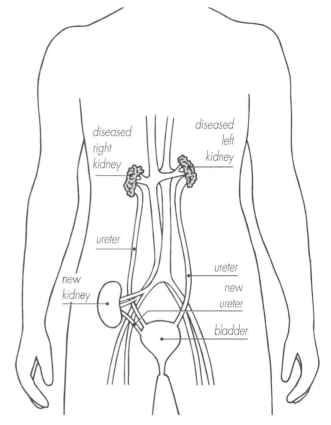

Figure 6.2: The transplant operation: placing of the transplanted kidney

abdomen, just above the groin (see Figure 6.2). The transplant kidney has its own artery (to take blood to it), vein (to take blood from it) and ureter (to take urine to the bladder).

The artery belonging to the new kidney is attached to the patient's main artery supplying blood to the leg on that side of the body. The vein belonging to the new kidney is attached to the main vein carrying blood from that leg. The transplant kidney's ureter is attached to the patient's own bladder.

A small plastic pipe (called a double J stent) is sometimes inserted into the ureter (see Figure 6.3) to help prevent the ureter from becoming blocked after the operation.

At the end of the operation, the patient's abdomen is closed with stitches.

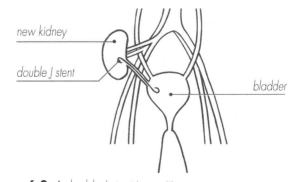

Figure 6.3: A double J stent in position

After the operation

The first few days after the operation are critical, and patients are monitored very closely. Particular attention is paid to blood pressure, fluid intake and urine output.

Most patients are able to drink and eat small amounts and also to sit out of bed the day after the operation.

Patients will have blood tests measured every day. This shows whether or not the transplant kidney is working. The amount of urine that the new kidney makes is not a reliable measure, as people who have just had a transplant may produce a large volume of urine that does not contain many toxins.

In about one-third of kidney transplant patients, the kidney does not produce any urine in the first few days after the operation. This does not mean that the transplant will never work. If the transplant does not work at the start, patients will need to continue dialysis and play a waiting game until the kidney starts working. Remember, a 'good transplant' is one that is working well after one year, not two weeks.

Patients will usually stay in hospital for about two weeks.

Follow up

After leaving hospital, kidney transplant patients will need to go to the clinic very frequently for many months, initially 2–3 times per week, then once a week, then once every two weeks, and so on. When the doctors are satisfied that the kidney is working well, the patient's appointments may be extended to once every three months or so.

It usually takes 3–6 months for patients who have had a kidney transplant to return to normal activities, including work. Transplant patients are recommended not to drive for at least one month after the operation. The function of the kidney, and the risk of infection, will not be affected by having sex. However, it is probably best not to resume sexual activity until about four weeks after leaving hospital.

Matching kidneys for transplants

For a kidney transplant to be successful, it is better that the blood and tissues of the new kidney are fairly similar (i.e. 'matched') to the patient's body. If the new kidney is not well matched, the patient's immune system (natural defence system) will be more likely to attack and reject it.

There are two things that are matched: the blood group and tissue type and these are checked for the donor kidney and the recipient of the transplant.

Blood group. Your blood group found by having a simple blood test. It is inherited from one of your parents. There are four blood groups.

- A
- B
- AB and
- O

Group O is the most common, followed by group A, then B then AB – except in Asian patients, in whom group B is more common than A.

Your blood group acts as a 'friendly face' for the body's cells, so they can be recognised as their own, and leave them alone. A person's immune system will attack any cells that have a foreign antigen. This means a patient can only normally be given a transplant kidney if the patient's and donor's blood groups are matched as follows:

Patient	Donor
Group O	Group O
Group A	Group A or Group O
Group B	Group B or Group O
Group AB	Any group (O, A, B, or AB)

Tissue type. Matching for tissue type is similar to matching for blood group. Again, the tissue type is found by a blood test. It shows a person's genetic make-up (a type of 'genetic fingerprint'). You have only one tissue type (just as you only have one blood group), but your tissue type is made up of six different tissue type characteristics.

There are three main parts of the tissue type; A, B and

DR. Everyone has two of each (one from each parent) making six in all.

So, for example, a tissue type could be A1/A2, B7/B8, DR2/DR3.

As there are so many possible tissue types, matching tissue types is a little more complicated than matching blood groups. However, the more pairs of tissue type that are the same for both patient and donor kidney, the better will be the chances that the transplant kidney will work.

Given the large number of tissue type possibilities, it is very unusual to get an exact match between a patient and donor. Most units will offer a transplant if the patient and donor have three or more of the six tissue type characteristics in common.

The better the match, the more likely it is that the body will accept the kidney 'as its own', and not try to reject it. This means that the kidney transplant is more likely to work well and keep you healthy in the long term

Unfortunately, it cannot be guaranteed that even a '6 out of 6' match will not be rejected. Tissue-type matching is less important for transplants from living donors where a 1 out of 6 match may be enough.

Where do kidneys for transplants come from?

Deceased donor transplants

A transplant kidney that has been removed from someone who has died is called a deceased donor transplant. About 65% of transplant kidneys in the UK come from this source and approximately 85% are still working after five years.

Brain stem death. Most deceased donors have been killed in car accidents or have died from a stroke, and have been on a life support machine (ventilator) in an intensive care unit. The ventilator is breathing for them. Their organs can be removed and donated after the person has been diagnosed 'brain dead'. This means the part of the brain called the brainstem, which controls breathing, has permanently stopped working. An individual who is brainstem dead cannot stay on a life support machine indefinitely, as their heart will stop relatively soon.

Deceased cardiac dead donors. Because of the shortage of donors, some kidney units are obtaining transplant kidneys from people who have died up to 30 minutes previously. These donors – called deceased cardiac dead (or asystolic) donors – are people who have died very suddenly, sometimes from a heart attack. Their hearts have stopped beating, and they are dead. However, they had not necessarily been put on a life support machine.

Deceased cardiac dead transplants do not always work immediately after the transplant operation and a period of dialysis may be needed. This does not normally affect the long-term results.

Patients who are offered a transplant can ask whether it is from a cardiac dead or brain dead donor. However, you are not told any other details about the donor.

After receiving a deceased donor kidney, patients may write to the donor's family, via the transplant co-ordinator, if they wish, but both donor and recipient remain anonymous.

If someone is on the national waiting list for a deceased donor kidney, they can still ask a relative, partner or friend to give them a kidney.

The transplant 'waiting list'

People who are suitable for a kidney transplant usually have to wait for a healthy kidney to be donated. Most living donated kidneys are organised via the patient and donor directly, with the support of the transplant team from the hospital.

For patients who opt for a deceased donor transplant, there is a national system that seeks to find the 'right' transplant organ for the 'right' patient. This is called the transplant waiting list. It is run by UK Blood and Transplant (UKBT), where the computer system compares patients' details (including blood group and tissue type) with those of deceased donor organs that become available.

The waiting list works on the basis of finding the 'right' dialysis patient for the 'right' kidney, when one becomes available. It does not work on a 'first-come, first-served' basis. So it is not really a waiting list, more of a register.

At present, not enough deceased donor kidneys are offered to meet the demand. Changes in seat-belt laws and improvements in medicine mean that fewer people now die from the accidents or illnesses that would have made them suitable donors.

If a person dies, and their family agree to donate the organs, surgeons remove the two kidneys. These kidneys are tested to make sure that they are healthy, and the blood group and tissue type are entered into the computer at UKBT.

The average waiting time for a deceased donor transplant kidney is about three years. This is an average, though, and will depend on the patient's blood group, tissue type and general health. A nationally agreed 'scoring system' decides where the kidneys go. It is based on a combination of blood group and tissue type matching, and the length of time the patient has been on the waiting list, and some other factors.

Even though it is as fair as it can be, some patients are disadvantaged. For example, people of Asian origin may wait longer. This is partly because Asian people tend to have different blood groups from white people, and there are fewer Asian donors. It is particularly important therefore for Asian patients to find a living donor in their family, as they may have to wait a very long time to get a deceased donor kidney in the UK.

It may sometimes be necessary to take a patient off the transplant list. This may be done, for example, if someone develops a serious infection or a heart problem, or if they need a major operation.

Any patient whose name is removed from the list should be told about the decision, and informed whether removal from the list is temporary or permanent. Patients who are unsure whether or not they are 'on the list' should ask their kidney doctor or nurse and then ask them for proof in writing.

Living donor transplants

Human beings do not need two kidneys to remain healthy. The loss of one kidney will not usually cause any harm to the donor, providing the other one is healthy and functioning.

Living donors can either be a blood relative of the recipient (mother, father, brother, sister, aunt, uncle, son or daughter) or unrelated to the recipient (husband, wife, friend or altruistic donor).

About 35% of transplants in the UK are from living donors and approximately 90% are still working after five years.

A transplant from a living donor can have many benefits. If someone is kind enough to donate a kidney, the whole transplant procedure will be planned, and both donor and recipient are usually well prepared for the operation. In some circumstances, the transplant may take place before you need to start dialysis. The transplant operation can also be planned on a date which is suitable for everyone involved, whereas deceased donor transplants often happen at very short notice.

However, there are risks with the procedure. As with any type of transplant, the new kidney may not work – in fact, 3% of living transplants are not working a year after the transplant operation. So it is worth considering the emotional aspects of living transplantation before embarking on the process. Both you and the donor need to talk about the possibility of complications following the operation, and how you might feel if the transplant doesn't work.

Most transplant units in the UK have a transplant co-ordinator whose main job is to organise living transplants. Anyone who is on the list for a deceased donor transplant can have a living donor transplant if they have a suitable donor.

Who can be a 'living donor'?

Almost anyone can donate a kidney to a loved one. The best donor is an identical twin, as the tissue type is identical – but that is very rare as you might imagine! If a kidney patient has a friend, partner or relative who is at least 16 years old, healthy, and willing to give them a kidney, the best advice is to ask them to speak to the transplant co-ordinator (or other senior nurse or doctor) at their unit.

The most suitable donor is usually a father, mother, brother, sister, son or daughter, but other more distant relatives may be suitable – uncle, aunt, nephew, niece, cousin, grandparent or grandchild. In fact, the donor does not necessarily have to be a blood relative. The patient's wife, husband, partner or close friend may also be suitable.

There are some situations where it would not be possible for a living person to donate a kidney. These include potential donors with:

- HIV or AIDS-related infection;
- hepatitis B or C infection;
- major heart or breathing problems;
- diabetes;
- significant kidney disease;
- cancer;
- very high blood pressure;
- a history of intravenous drug abuse;
- extreme obesity;
- pregnancy;
- only one kidney;
- evidence of financial or non-financial coercion;
- inability to give informed consent; or
- age below 16 years.

In addition, doctors would think very seriously before allowing anyone to donate a kidney if any of the following applied:

- age over 70 years;
- age below 18 years;
- intellectual impairment but able to give informed consent;
- mild obesity;
- family history of diabetes;
- psychiatric disorders; or
- mild high blood pressure (i.e. needing more than one blood pressure tablet).

Which donor is best?

If more than one person is a suitable donor, it can be difficult to decide which one to accept a kidney from. But if a patient has a parent and a brother or sister, both of whom are willing (and able) to donate, it might be 'better' to accept the kidney from the parent now, and then 'keep' the sibling's kidney for later in life, if the first transplant ever fails.

Who will do the asking?

It is up to kidney patients to ask their friends or family to see if they are willing to donate a kidney. Doctors will not usually ask a patient's loved ones for them, but they will talk to anybody who is willing to donate a kidney.

Tests for the donor

The potential transplant donor will first be tested for their blood group and tissue type. Usually, if the patient's blood group and the donor's blood group are not compatible (according to the rules outlined), the transplant is unlikely to go ahead.

Some transplant units have introduced a technique called antibody incompatible transplants which makes it possible for a patient to have a successful transplant when a donor is in the 'wrong' group (see below for more details). If your transplant unit does not do this type of transplant, you can be referred to another transplant centre.

If the test is OK, blood samples will be taken to test the donor's liver and kidney function. If these prove satisfactory, the next stage of the screening process can then go ahead.

The donor will need to have a thorough medical examination. This is usually done by two separate doctors – a kidney doctor (usually a different one from the doctor responsible for the patient), and the surgeon who will perform the operation. The doctors will check to make sure that the donor has a normal blood pressure.

In some cases, the transplant may still go ahead, even if the donor has high blood pressure, just as long as it is well controlled using only one type of blood pressure tablet.

An ultrasound scan will then be used to make sure that the donor has two kidneys, and that both are working equally well.

The potential donor will also have an ECG (a heart trace) and a chest X-ray to ensure there are no problems with their heart or breathing. They may also be given an exercise tolerance test to see how their heart reacts during exercise. Blood tests will be carried out for infections such as HIV and hepatitis B and C.

In addition, there will be a cross-match test between donor and recipient. If the cross-match is negative, this means the transplant work-up can continue. However, sometimes an antibody incompatible transplant can get around this problem.

Most units will also carry out a psychological assessment of both donor and recipient. This is to make sure that both are happy about the procedure, and the effects it may have on them and their families. The psychologist will make sure that both people are able to cope if the transplant fails or if anything happens to either the donor or the recipient.

Finally, to help the surgeons decide which kidney (left or right) to remove, the blood vessels to each kidney must be examined using CT scans.

Paired donation

In 2004 the Human Tissue Act introduced a system called 'pairing' donated kidneys.

If a person who needs a new kidney has a family member or close friend who is willing to donate a kidney to them, but who has an incompatible blood group or tissue type, paired donation may be possible.

Paired donation allows both kidney donors and recipients to be matched up.

Local transplant centres will assess whether people are suitable to be put forward for paired donation. If so, their details will be put on to a national register where they can be matched to a compatible pair. Donor and recipient operations are planned to happen at the same time so that organs can be exchanged at the same time.

Antibody incompatible transplants

Some kidney patients have high levels of antibody to a potential donor. The patient may also have the 'wrong' (i.e. incompatible) blood group, tissue type, or both. Usually, if a kidney that is incompatible was transplanted, the recipient's body would reject the kidney. A technique called antibody incompatible transplant is offered to patients in some transplant centres in the UK. It involves using immunosuppression medicines that are stronger than normal; using a dialysis-like process called plasmapharesis and other strong drugs.

This procedure has proved to be very successful in allowing more patients to have a kidney donated from someone who isn't a good match for either blood group or tissue type.

Altruistic donation

The 2006 Human Tissue Act made it legal for a person to donate a kidney to a stranger. This is called an altruistic donation. An altruistic donor must go through the same checks as a donor who is known to the recipient.

Although altruistic kidney donation is quite rare, it is becoming more popular. In 2007 only six people donated a kidney – however, more than 130 altruistic donations were received in 2018.

In some parts of the UK, the altruistic donor has been linked to a 'paired' donation scheme.

Buying and selling organs

In the UK, it is illegal to buy or sell kidneys for transplant. There must be no pressure put on any potential donor to donate, or recipient to accept. Even though it is illegal to offer payment to enable the live transplant to take place, it is legal for the donor to be repaid reasonable costs incurred due to travelling or loss of earnings.

How long does it take to get a living donor transplant?

The length of time it takes to prepare the donor and recipient for a living donor kidney transplant can vary. On average, it can take around 3–6 months.

It is important that the donor allows for time off work before the transplant as well as after, so that the relevant tests can all be done.

Pre-emptive transplants

A pre-emptive transplant is when kidney transplant operation is carried out before the patient needs to start dialysis. About 10% of patients have a kidney transplant as their first treatment rather than dialysis, and this number is growing every year. Most people who have a pre-emptive transplant will have the operation about six months before they are likely to need dialysis.

Some kidney units are undoubtedly better at organising pre-emptive transplants than others. On average about 40% of patients are put on the list for a transplant before they start dialysis. This varies across the UK.

The timing of a pre-emptive transplant may be difficult to get right. You don't want to have the kidney transplant too early, before you really need treatment, and have all of the problems with the medications as well as 'using up' the life of the kidney. However, you don't want to wait too long, as you may have unpleasant symptoms.

You can ask the doctors, nurses or managers how many pre-emptive transplants are done in your transplanting unit. You can also find out this information on the NHS Blood and Transplant website. You will find that performance does vary quite considerably around the UK.

For most patients, the possibility of obtaining a transplant kidney from a living donor will be the best chance of having a transplant operation before dialysis is needed.

Removing the kidney from the donor

There are two ways a live kidney can be donated, either by open surgery, or laparoscopically (using keyhole surgery). The removal of a kidney is called a nephrectomy.

1 **Open nephrectomy.** Open surgery is the most common method of removing the kidney. The surgeon makes a cut from the middle point of the side of the chest to the side of the abdomen. Part of a rib may also need to be removed. This method leaves a much larger scar than keyhole surgery. It also takes longer for the donor to recover after the operation.

2 **Laparoscopic nephrectomy.** Some kidney units remove the kidney using keyhole surgery. A small cut is made above the pubic hairline. The kidney is removed with the help of a small camera that helps the surgeon to see inside the body without cutting the patient right open. The benefit of this procedure is that the patient has a smaller scar and a quicker recovery time.

Whichever method is used to remove the kidney, the surgeon also removes the blood vessels and tubes surrounding the kidney, as they will be used for the recipient.

If the kidney is removed using laparoscopic nephrectomy, the donor will be in hospital for about 3–5 days, but after open surgery this could be 6–9 days.

How soon the donor returns to work will depend on the type of work and their general fitness before the operation. If the work is physically demanding, the donor will probably need a longer recovery time than someone who has sedentary work.

Risks to the donor

Although any surgery carries a small risk, the risks to a healthy donor should be minimal if all the pre-operative tests have been carried out.

Anyone who donates a kidney will be seen regularly after the operation. Most units recommend kidney donors should be seen by a kidney specialist every year for life.

There is some evidence to suggest that kidney donors

live longer than other people on average – although why this is the case is not clear.

There will be some pain and discomfort after the operation, which should get better after a few days. One in 25 patients has long-term pain in the site of the wound. This can usually be controlled by injections given from time to time.

Some donors may experience protein in their urine (proteinuria) after the operation.

There is a 1 in 3,000 chance of the donor dying during or after the operation. This is similar to the risk of any major operation. A more common and major problem of donating a kidney to a loved one is the potential emotional upset if a living donor transplant fails at an early stage.

How long will a transplant last?

A kidney transplant from a live donor is likely to function for longer than a deceased donor kidney. On average 90% of living donor transplants are still working after five years compared to 85% of transplants from deceased donors.

One reason that it is thought that living donor transplants last longer than deceased donor transplants is that the donors are carefully screened before the operation. Any diseases that might affect the kidneys, such as high blood pressure or diabetes, are checked for. If evidence of them is found, the donor's kidneys won't be used. The donor's kidneys are also checked to make sure that they function perfectly, and are not likely to fail in the future.

Another factor that might improve the outcome is the time in which the kidney is outside a human body after it has been removed from the donor – called the cold ischaemia time. This is less than one hour for a live transplant, but 12–36 hours (the average is 20 hours) for a deceased donor transplant.

There is also some evidence to suggest that the recipient of a living donor transplant is more likely to take the medication required after the transplant, perhaps because the recipient feels more of a responsibility towards the new kidney.

Life expectancy

Having a kidney transplant may also improve a patient's life expectancy: 99% of patients who have a living donor transplant are still alive a year after the operation, and 95% are still alive five years after the operation.

The results are not quite so good for deceased donor transplants with 96% of patients still being alive a year after the operation and 89% being alive five years after the operation. This compares to about 70% of patients who are still alive one year of starting dialysis and 50% who are living five years after starting dialysis. This is a not an entirely fair comparison, as transplant patients are generally younger than many people on dialysis and so would be expected to live longer.

New developments and the future

There has always been a lot of interest in research in the area of kidney transplantation. Much of the research to date has focused on anti-rejection drugs; however, there are other exciting developments.

Robotic arm laparoscopic kidney transplants

Some surgeons are pioneering a new method of kidney transplants using a laparoscope (a tiny camera inserted into the body) and a robotic device. The advantage of this method is that the hole made for the operation is only about 2 inches, and therefore the scar is very small. The robot is used to stitch the blood vessels from the donor kidney to the patient's blood vessels.

This method is most useful for people who are very overweight. This is because the usual operation for kidney transplants doesn't always work as well for obese patients and there is a very high risk that the operation scar will become infected after the operation.

Stem cell therapy

There has been a lot of publicity about a new technique called regenerative medicine or stem cell therapy. This is where organs, including limbs, livers, skin and heart tissues are grown from stem cells in a laboratory. However, while it has been possible to grow the cells, actually getting a functioning organ has been much more difficult.

Recently, researchers in Japan reported that they grew fully functioning kidneys in the lab, and when transplanted into pigs and rats, thoes kidneys produced urine.

Unfortunately, the prospect of doing trials of this technique in humans is still a long way in the future.

Gene therapy

There has been research looking into using the kidneys of pigs for human transplantation for many years. Called xenotransplantation, the science has always been slowed down by the huge problems of rejection of a pig's kidney from the human recipient. However, as recently as 2015, scientists in the USA have been changing the genes in pigs before the organ is transplanted. Experiments are in the early phase and have so far only been carried out using pig kidneys in a baboon.

KEY FACTS

1 Transplant kidneys can be donated by a deceased donor or a living donor.

2 It is possible to have a transplant before dialysis is started.

3 A transplant operation lasts about 2 hours, and the patient will need to stay in hospital for about two weeks after the operation.

4 About a third of transplanted kidneys do not work right away. Sometimes this means the patient will need to have dialysis until it does start to work.

5 Acute rejection of the kidney is usually fairly easy to treat.

6 Patients have to take immunosuppressant drugs daily to prevent their body rejecting a transplant. Not taking them correctly can lead to loss of the kidney. However, these drugs do have side effects.

7 A transplant does not always last for ever. Transplants from living relatives last longest.

8 If a transplant fails, you can go back onto dialysis. Most people can go on to have another transplant.

9 It is important to keep as fit as possible after a transplant. For example, don't smoke, try to keep your weight down, monitor your blood pressure, cholesterol levels and (if you have diabetes) your blood sugar.

10 If you have had a transplant, you will be at greater risk than other people of developing skin cancer, so be extra careful about protecting your skin from the sun. You will also have an increased risk of developing lymphoma, which can sometimes be fatal.

7 DRUG TREATMENTS FOR BLOOD PRESSURE, ANAEMIA AND BONES

This chapter looks at the treatments that people with kidney failure need to manage their blood pressure, anaemia and bones. It explains why these are necessary, how they help to manage your symptoms and what part you can play in staying well.

Introduction
The kidneys have many different functions in the body. These are described in detail in Chapter 1. Along with making urine, which allows wastes and excess fluid to be removed from the body, the kidneys also:
- help to control blood pressure;
- help to control the manufacture of red blood cells;
- help to keep the bones strong and healthy.

Treatment with dialysis is only able to help remove excess fluid and wastes. There is therefore a need to replace these other kidney functions and this is usually done by using a variety of different medicines. These medicines are taken in the form of tablets or injections.

Controlling high blood pressure
The term 'blood pressure' means the pressure of the blood on the artery walls which are the tubes that carry blood around the body. This pressure goes up and down as the heart continuously squeezes and relaxes to pump blood around the body. The kidneys play an important role in keeping the blood pressure stable. So, when the kidneys stop working, many patients find they have problems controlling their blood pressure. It is more likely that people with kidney failure will have high blood pressure (rather than low blood pressure).

How is high blood pressure treated?
There are a number of ways that high blood pressure can be controlled. The first is by making improvements to your lifestyle by taking regular exercise, eating healthily so as not to become overweight and by limiting the amount of salt you eat, and by not smoking. These are all discussed in detail in Chapter 12. Here we focus on the medicines that can be used to reduce your blood pressure.

Drugs for high blood pressure
There are a number of different drugs that are used to manage high blood pressure. Those that:
- act directly on the kidney to lower the blood pressure (ACE inhibitor drugs and ARB drugs);
- widen the arteries (vasodilators);
- remove excess water from the body (loop diuretics and thiazide drugs);

- act on the body's blood pressure control signals (centrally acting antihypertensive drugs).

Drugs that act directly on the kidney

There are two types of drugs that act directly on the kidney to control blood pressure. These are known as ACEis and ARBs.

ACEi (or ACE inhibitors) are drugs such as captopril, enalapril, lisinopril, perindopril and ramipril. ACE stands for Angiotensin Converting Enzyme and ACE inhibitors work by stopping your body from producing a chemical called angiotensin 2. This chemical is produced by your kidneys and lungs working together. When angiotensin 2 enters your bloodstream your blood vessels become narrower. This gives your blood less space to move in, which raises your blood pressure. So if the body doesn't produce as much angiotensin 2, the blood vessels will stay wider.

ARBs (or Angiotensin Receptor Blockers) are drugs such as candesartan, irbesartan, losartan and telmisartan. These drugs work in a similar way to ACE inhibitors.

Both of these types of drugs also work within the kidneys themselves and are therefore used very often in people with kidney disease. The kidneys are made up of thousands of filters called glomeruli. They have a blood vessel that feeds into them from the heart and one that passes the blood back to the rest of the body toward the heart. In kidney disease the pressure inside these filters can rise and cause damage. These drugs relax or widen the outflow blood vessel, reducing the pressure in the filter and reducing the risk of damage. For more information on what your kidneys do, take a visit to www.thinkkidneys.nhs.uk/campaign and have a look at the animation.

Vasodilators

Blood pressure tablets called vasodilators lower the blood pressure by causing the arteries to widen. There are several different types of vasodilator drug.

Alpha blockers (e.g. doxazosin, prazosin and terazosin). Alpha receptors are chemicals found in the muscles around the blood vessels and they make the muscle tighten up. This causes the blood vessels to become smaller which makes the blood pressure higher. Alpha-blockers stop this from happening, so the muscles in the blood vessels stay relaxed and blood can flow more easily, thereby lowering your blood pressure.

Calcium channel blockers (e.g. amlodipine, diltiazem, felodipine and nifedipine). Calcium is another substance that acts to narrow the blood vessels and these drugs stop calcium from being able to get into the muscles. Eating grapefruit or drinking grapefruit juice when you take these drugs can cause side effects.

Diuretics (water tablets)

If someone has fluid overload, their blood pressure will increase. This is because their blood contains more water than normal, which increases the pressure on the blood vessels. Correcting fluid overload (see Chapter 11) with diuretics (water tablets) or dialysis will reduce the blood pressure. Eating a lot of salty foods and adding extra salt to meals makes people thirsty and leads to them drinking more. So, people with kidney failure should cut down on salt as well as fluid.

In fact diuretics are misnamed – they actually make the kidneys pass more salt and the water comes along with the salt. Remember – salt and water go together (see Chapter 11).

There are two main types of diuretics; loop diuretics and thiazides.

Loop diuretics work directly on the part of the kidney that controls the amount of water the body removes in the urine, known as the loop of Henle. So when you take a loop diuretic, you will pass more urine and therefore more salt and water will be removed from the body. Even though people with kidney failure don't produce much urine, loop diuretics can still work and can be used in people on dialysis although the dose needs to be higher.

Thiazides will also make you pass more urine and so lower the blood pressure, although exactly how they work is not known.

Other drugs – beta blockers and centrally acting drugs (e.g. moxonidine)

Beta blockers reduce the force of contraction and the heart rate (the number of heart beats per minute) which lowers the blood pressure. Commonly used beta- blockers are atenolol, bisoprolol, carvedilol, labetalol, metoprolol and propranolol.

Other tablets that may be given for high blood pressure work on the whole body. These drugs are hydralazine, methyldopa, minoxidil and moxonidine. Moxonidine is a drug that stimulates chemicals in the brain called imidazoline receptors. This reduces the signals that are sent from the brain to the blood vessels which usually cause them to contract and narrow. Therefore, when these signals are stopped or reduced the blood vessels are allowed to relax and widen. This increases the amount of space in the blood vessels and so decreases the pressure inside them. This lowers blood pressure.

Treatments for anaemia

Many patients with kidney failure have a condition called anaemia. This means that they have a lack of red blood cells in their body. Blood cells are produced in the bone marrow, the 'runny' bit in the middle of the bones. An important 'extra' function of the kidneys is to help control the manufacture of red blood cells in the bone marrow.

Composition of the blood

Blood is made up of two parts: a liquid part and a more solid part (see Figure 7.1). The liquid part is called plasma. About 60% of the blood is plasma, and it is mainly water. The other 40% of the blood is made up of blood cells, which are so tiny that they can only be seen through a microscope. There are various different types of cells: red cells (which carry oxygen around the body), white cells

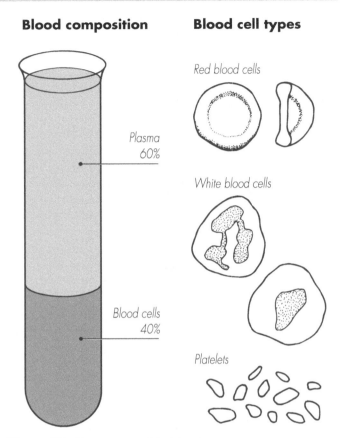

Figure 7.1: Composition of the blood

(which fight infection) and platelets (which help the blood to clot). Most of the blood cells are red cells. It is these cells that give the blood its red colour. You have about 5 billion red cells in one drop of blood.

What is anaemia?

Anaemia is the term for a lack of red blood cells in the body. The main symptoms are tiredness, shortness of breath, pale skin, poor appetite, irritability and low sex drive. Anaemia is the main reason why people with kidney failure feel weak and tired.

Red blood cells are needed to carry oxygen around the body. Oxygen enters the lungs when we breathe in. From the lungs, oxygen is taken around the body in the blood. Each red blood cell contains a substance called haemoglobin. It is the haemoglobin that carries oxygen around the body.

To help the haemoglobin to work properly, iron is needed. Iron in the blood is also known as ferritin. The doctors measure both the haemoglobin and the ferritin levels in people with kidney failure.

Haemoglobin (or 'Hb') levels in healthy people are between 120–170 g/L (grams of haemoglobin per litre of blood). However, if you have kidney failure the target level Hb is between 100–120 g/L.

Ferritin levels should be between 200 and 500 µg/L (micrograms per litre of blood).

Why do people with kidney failure develop anaemia?

The kidneys manage the production of red blood cells in the bone marrow. To do this, they make a substance called erythropoietin (EPO) which is a hormone (a chemical messenger). EPO travels in the blood from the kidneys to the bone marrow, where it constantly reminds the bone marrow to keep producing red cells. When someone has kidney failure, the kidneys usually make less EPO than normal. So the bone marrow makes fewer red cells. As a result, anaemia develops, and the patient becomes weak and tired.

Some patients with kidney failure develop anaemia even though their EPO level is normal. This probably means that their bone marrow has a problem reacting to EPO, or that there is not enough iron in the blood. Although a lack of EPO is the main cause of anaemia in people with kidney failure, other things may contribute. For example, red blood cells do not live as long as normal (120 days) in people with kidney failure, and so must be replaced more often. Also, blood may be lost during haemodialysis, or through frequent blood tests.

Treatment for anaemia for people with kidney failure

Before the introduction of EPO Stimulating Agent (ESA) injections, blood transfusions were the only treatment for anaemia in kidney patients. Many patients had to have transfusions every couple of months, since each transfusion could improve anaemia for a few weeks only. Blood transfusions can cause serious problems for patients on dialysis. These include fluid overload and the storage of excess iron in the liver (which can lead to liver failure). Another problem is that whenever a transfusion of blood is received, the body produces substances called antibodies. These antibodies stay in the blood for years and can cause problems if the patient is then given a transplant. The antibodies can attack (and cause the body to reject) the new kidney. For all of these reasons blood transfusions are not the best treatment for kidney patients and are avoided.

Blood transfusions are still sometimes needed by kidney patients – for example, after severe bleeding.

ESA

Erythropoiesis stimulating agent (ESA) medicines are man-made versions of erythropoietin or other substances that stimulate the bone marrow to produce red cells. An ESA is generally given in the form of an injection under the skin (called a subcutaneous injection). Some ESAs (called epoetin alfa and epoetin beta), are given one, two or three times a week. Other types of ESA (such as darbepoetin alfa) last much longer and so only need to be given every few weeks.

Many patients give their own injections, particularly those on home dialysis such as PD or Home HD, although a nurse can give the injection if necessary. The aim of the treatment is to raise the Hb level in the blood to between 100 and 120 g/L. Without this treatment, most patients with kidney failure would have an Hb between 60 and 80 g/L and need lots of blood transfusions.

A patient's response to an ESA depends on how much

they are given and the levels of iron they have in their blood. The higher or more frequent the dose, the higher the patient's blood Hb level will go.

There is no point, however, in making the Hb go above 120 g/L – the patient will feel no better. In fact, problems may occur if the Hb goes over 140 g/L. For example, a fistula may clot and stop working. So, the target Hb is 100–120 g/L in most patients, and they should take ESAs only as prescribed.

Who needs an ESA?

Patients who are on dialysis – either PD (see Chapter 4) or haemodialysis (see Chapter 5) – often need an ESA. In fact about 90% of people who are on haemodialysis and 70% of people who are on PD take an ESA. There are fewer patients on PD taking an ESA because PD patients tend to have less of a problem with anaemia. If they are prescribed an ESA, they usually need a lower dose.

For most patients, anaemia actually begins long before they need to start dialysis. Therefore many patients with CKD are given ESAs before the start of dialysis, in the pre-dialysis period. Transplant patients may also need an ESA if their Hb falls below 100 g/L, especially if the transplant is failing, as anaemia often returns at this time.

Are there any side effects?

The only common side effect of ESAs is worsening of high blood pressure. If the blood pressure does increase, more blood pressure tablets may need to be taken. A combination of an ESA and high blood pressure can sometimes cause epileptic fits, but this problem can usually be prevented by treating the high blood pressure.

Iron supplements

Iron deficiency is a common problem for people with kidney failure. If there isn't enough iron in the blood, the ESA won't work. Blood ferritin levels provide a guide to the amount of iron in the body and the value should be at least 200 micrograms per litre.

If absolute iron deficiency is discovered, the doctors should investigate why the patient lacks iron. One important cause could be bleeding (that may not have been noticed by the patient) from somewhere in the bowel.

Most people with kidney failure are treated with iron either as tablets (usually a type called ferrous sulphate) or as injections. Which type is used depends on the degree of kidney failure, the other medicines that someone might need and some other factors. For example, iron given as a drip is felt to be more effective than tablets for someone on dialysis.

Anaemia and transplantation

After a kidney transplant, the new kidney will start making EPO for the patient and the problem of anaemia usually goes away. Injections of an ESA will then no longer be needed. However, if the transplanted kidney ever fails, anaemia will usually return, and ESA injections may be needed again.

Treatment for bone problems

Healthy kidneys keep bones strong by balancing calcium, phosphate and vitamin D in the body. People think that our bones are lumps of rock that hold us up but in fact they are very active organs. To cope with the stresses and strains of life they are consistently being broken down on a microscopic level and then rebuilt. When the kidneys don't work well, bones can become damaged. This can be due to a failure to remake or rebuild the bones – a job done by activated vitamin D and needing calcium. Or it can be due to the bones becoming overactive, being broken down quicker than they can be made. This process is driven by a hormone called parathyroid hormone or parathormone (PTH), produced by four glands that sit behind the thyroid gland at the front of your neck. High levels of PTH can result from a lack of activated vitamin D and also by high levels of phosphate in the blood. Phosphate concentrations are regulated by the kidneys.

When kidney function declines, the levels of phosphate in the blood rise. This makes the body produce more PTH to help the kidneys get rid of the excess phosphate. So that is why in the early stages there are no changes in the simple blood tests. The body's mechanisms adapt to try and make up for the reduced kidney function. But as kidney function falls further the body can no longer compensate and problems then develop.

So calcium and phosphate are the building blocks of the bones with the main reserve in the bones and a small amount that is accessible in the blood. Vitamin D is the remaker of bones and PTH breaks them down to allow them to be remade. Just to finish with this complex story (and there is a lot more to it) vitamin D also raises calcium in other ways and makes the parathyroid glands reduce the amount of PTH they produce.

Development of renal bone disease

Renal bone disease can start in the early stages of kidney disease, a long time before dialysis or a transplant is needed. Standard blood tests, done when people have Stage 2 or 3 of kidney disease (CKD Stage 2 or 3) may show low calcium concentrations and high concentrations of phosphate but these become more common as kidney function reduces. In general, only the measurement of calcium and phosphate is needed before you reach CKD Stage 4. Once someone reaches CKD Stage 4, PTH concentrations will be measured on a regular basis and in some people vitamin D levels will also be measured.

What is renal bone disease and how does it happen?

Renal bone disease is a term used to describe the bone problems associated with kidney disease and kidney failure. In fact renal bone disease is more than one thing. There are a number of factors that lead to renal bone disease. In addition, it is now thought that the problems seen that lead to renal bone disease have wider harmful effects on the heart, heart valves and blood vessels of someone with kidney problems. It is for all these reasons that it is important to control renal bone disease.

Low levels of activated vitamin D in the blood. Vitamin D is needed to help the calcium we eat to be used to strengthen the bones. Vitamin D is found in some food, especially margarine and butter. However, most of our vitamin D come through our skin from the sunlight. Unfortunately, the body can't use vitamin D directly from food or sunshine unless it is changed. The kidneys do the job of changing vitamin D so that the body can use it to help the calcium work properly. It is quite easy to provide usable vitamin D as tablets or injections.

High phosphate levels in the blood. Phosphate is another mineral that keeps bones strong. Foods that contain phosphate are dairy products (milk, cheese and yoghurt), nuts and meat. Like calcium, phosphate is stored in the body in the bones. The kidneys normally help to keep the right amount in the body – not too much, not too little. When kidneys stop working, phosphate builds up in the blood.

Low calcium levels in the blood. Calcium is a mineral that strengthens the bones. It comes from food, especially dairy products (milk, cheese and yoghurt), eggs and green vegetables. In our bodies, calcium is stored in the bones.

Healthy kidneys help to keep the right amount of calcium in the bones. In people with kidney failure, calcium drains out of the bones and is lost from the body. We can see if this has happened by measuring the concentration of calcium in the blood.

Parathyroid hormone and kidney failure

Parathyroid hormone (PTH) is a substance made by four tiny glands called the parathyroid glands. These glands are at the front of the neck (see Figure 7.2).

Normally the parathyroid glands make PTH when the amount of calcium in the blood is too low or the levels of activated vitamin D fall. PTH then allows calcium to be taken out of the bones so that the amount of calcium in the blood gets back to normal. If the PTH concentration rises above normal the bones may become weak as they become thin. This is called 'secondary hyperparathyroidism' because it is not a problem caused directly by the glands themselves.

Sometimes, if this process is not treated, it is difficult to stop the parathyroid gland from making lots of PTH. The glands are now in overdrive and the calcium level can now be high. This is called 'tertiary hyperparathyroidism'.

And yes, there is a 'primary hyperparathyroidism' where the glands become overactive on their own. But that is another story.

For more details about the correct levels of calcium, phosphate, vitamin D and parathyroid hormone in the body, see Chapter 13.

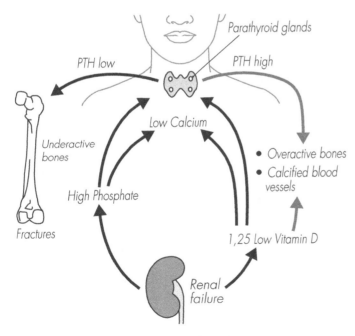

Figure 7.2: Secondary hyperparathyroidism

A combination of causes

Any one of these causes can lead to problems. Each of the causes tends to have a 'knock-on' effect, worsening the other two. For example, a high phosphate level will lower the calcium level, and vice versa. Keeping the balance isn't easy and so the doctors and nurses will check the blood levels regularly. It is important to make sure the calcium, phosphate, vitamin D and PTH are kept in control.

How is renal bone disease monitored?

Measuring the levels of calcium and phosphate in a kidney patient's blood can help tell what is happening in the bones at the time of the test. However, these levels cannot tell what the future health of the bones will be. The best way to know if renal bone disease will happen in the future is to measure the amount of PTH in the blood. On occasion, vitamin D levels may also be measured, especially if people are at risk of being short of vitamin D for other reasons.

How is renal bone disease treated?

Treatment for renal bone disease is monitored by trying to keep the concentrations of calcium, phosphate and PTH in suitable ranges. These ranges are not the same as the normal values for the general population and are set out in guidance from NICE and professional groups such as the Renal Association. Treatment for bone disease can be by changing the diet and by using drugs. For some people, an operation to remove the parathyroid gland may be needed.

Keep phosphate levels low

In the early stages of kidney failure, a diet with reduced phosphate may be helpful. Certain foods (e.g. dairy products) are high in phosphate and a dietitian will provide advice on what sort of diet to follow. As things progress, tablets can be used to bind the phosphate in the food. Exactly what time you take these tablets is different for each type of 'phosphate binder', so ask your dietitian. The tablets bind with the phosphate to stop the body from absorbing it. Phosphate binders work best when they are taken with food, and not at the same time as iron tablets. So taking the binders without a meal will give all of the side effects without any benefit. Forgetting to take the binders at the time of a meal will result in higher phosphate levels.

There are many types of phosphate binders – some contain calcium, some do not. At this time NICE recommends starting with a calcium-containing phosphate binder, changing to an alternative if there are problems. See Chapter 14 for more details on NICE Guidelines.

Unfortunately most types of dialysis do not remove very much phosphate. Many patients therefore need more treatment to control the phosphate level. However, 'High Dose Haemodialysis (HD)' seems to be very good at phosphate removal and many patients who have High Dose HD do not have high phosphate levels.

In some cases, the phosphate concentration is not high because of what is being eaten, but because the bones are overactive due to very high levels of PTH. In this case, reducing the PTH concentration will help.

Keep calcium levels normal

A diet to raise calcium concentrations is not usually very effective. A low calcium level normally means the person needs more vitamin D. So, calcium levels are raised by treatment with special 'active' vitamin D.

Sometimes, the calcium level can get too high, generally as a side effect of some types of phosphate binders or vitamin D tablets. This can be dangerous because the calcium builds up in the veins, arteries and around the heart making it difficult for blood to flow around the body. It is normally easily treated by changing the tablets.

Calcium concentrations can also be affected by the concentration of calcium in the dialysis solutions used in both haemodialysis and peritoneal dialysis. This can be adjusted by your renal team.

Low calcium levels can be the result of using cinacalcet to lower PTH production. See below for more information.

Make sure there is enough vitamin D

In a few patients, renal bone disease continues to be a problem even when the blood calcium and phosphate levels are brought under control. Treatment with 'active' vitamin D is then needed. This can be with calcitriol, alfacalcidol, or paricalcitol. PD patients receive vitamin D in the form of a tablet. Haemodialysis patients receive it either as tablet, or occasionally as an injection given during dialysis.

Control the parathyroid hormone (PTH)

In most patients, correcting the blood levels of calcium, phosphate and vitamin D is enough to control renal bone disease, and cause PTH levels to fall. In a few patients, however, this is not enough, and blood PTH levels continue to rise. When the PTH is extremely high more treatment is required to try to get it under control. This can be done by using a drug called cinacalcet or by having an operation to remove the parathyroid glands. This operation is called a parathyroidectomy.

If high PTH levels are not treated, the blood vessels (especially those that supply blood to the heart) can become 'furred up' with calcium, which can be very dangerous. Calcium may also build up in the eyes (making them red and itchy) or in the skin (which can cause parts of the skin to go black and die).

Transplants and renal bone disease

If a patient receives a transplant and the new kidney works well, the blood levels of calcium, phosphate, vitamin D and PTH will usually return to normal, or near normal. Renal bone disease then improves, although it never really goes away completely.

KEY FACTS

1 High blood pressure, anaemia and weak bones are very common in people with kidney failure.

2 High blood pressure can be controlled by removing fluid from your body and by taking blood pressure tablets.

3 Too much salt in the diet may make the blood pressure higher.

4 Anaemia is the main reason why dialysis patients are weak and tired.

5 Anaemia is treated with injections of substances called erythropoietin stimulating agents (ESAs).

6 ESAs are very good at controlling symptoms and giving you more energy. You should only stop taking them or miss a dose if your kidney doctor tells you to.

7 Renal bone disease is a major complication of kidney failure. Without treatment, it causes bone pain and fractures, and may also affect your heart and blood vessels.

8 Renal bone disease is caused by disorders of PTH, calcium, vitamin D, and phosphate.

9 Eating the right types of food and taking the tablets your doctor prescribes usually helps bone problems.

8 EATING WELL AND EXERCISING

This chapter explains why it is important for people with kidney failure to look after their general health by eating well and taking regular exercise. It describes the different dietary advice that is likely to be given as the treatments change. There is also some helpful advice about the types of exercise that are safest, depending on your type of treatment.

Introduction

Keeping generally fit by eating well and taking regular exercise is just as important for people who have kidney failure as it is for anyone else. You may find that the advice about what is best for you to eat changes over time. The reason is that people's dietary needs change as their kidney problems change. So, just as drug therapy and other treatments may need to be altered, diet may also need to be altered to stay in line.

Advice about taking regular exercise is unlikely to change, although there may be some different points to think about depending on what type of treatment you have.

Healthy eating guidelines

People with kidney failure – whether pre-dialysis, on dialysis or with a transplant – are advised to follow 'healthy eating guidelines'. These guidelines are:
- eat a varied diet;
- include some high-fibre foods (such as wholemeal bread and cereals);
- eat only moderate amounts of fats (which should be mainly polyunsaturated); and
- avoid adding 'extra' salt to foods, particularly if you have high blood pressure.

What is 'nutritional status'?

The term 'nutritional status' is used to describe how well-nourished we are. A person with a poor nutritional status may not be getting enough of the right kinds of food.

Unfortunately, there is no easy way to measure nutritional status. It can't be done by a simple blood test. Therefore it is usually assessed by:
- asking how the person is feeling in general;
- asking about the person's diet (perhaps including asking them to keep a record for a while of everything they eat and drink);
- measuring the size of the person's muscles;
- monitoring their body weight;
- measuring the level of albumin (a type of protein) in the blood. A low level of albumin is linked to malnutrition but is not a very accurate measure.

Protein

Protein is an essential nutrient, which helps the body to grow, build muscles, and to repair any damage. Most of the protein we eat comes from meat, fish, dairy products and pulses (such as beans and lentils). Everyone – including people with kidney failure – must eat the right amount of protein to avoid serious nutritional problems.

When protein is eaten, it is digested and used by the body. It is used to build muscles and repair damaged tissues but during this process, waste products are produced. One of these wastes is called urea. Healthy kidneys are quite good at getting rid of urea and other wastes from the blood. However, as kidney failure develops, the kidneys become less able to remove wastes from the blood.

This means that eating a lot of protein when you have kidney failure can cause the level of urea in the blood to get higher. Even so, this does not mean that people with kidney failure should stop eating protein because it is a very important nutrient.

Protein/energy supplements

Specialist protein and/or energy supplements can be helpful if a kidney patient is not eating enough. These supplements are very good and supply varying amounts of protein and energy depending on what is needed. They are available on prescription, and hospital dietitians can ask their patients' GPs to prescribe them.

The protein and energy supplements that you can buy from a health food shop or sports shop should not be taken by people with kidney failure unless the dietitian has given this specific advice.

Phosphate and calcium

Phosphate and calcium are two minerals that affect the health of the bones. When a person has kidney failure, the calcium level in their body tends to be too low, and their phosphate level too high. This puts them at risk of bone problems, due to a condition called renal bone disease.

Treatment for kidney patients therefore aims to raise blood calcium levels and also to lower blood phosphate levels. Both these aims can often be achieved by:

- reducing the phosphate content of your diet;
- getting enough dialysis if this has been started; and
- using a phosphate binder (calcium carbonate, e.g. Calcichew) taken as tablets with meals.

Phosphate binders stick onto the phosphate that is part of the food you eat and stop the body from absorbing it. Phosphate binders work best when they are taken at the right time and not at the same time as iron tablets. The timing of the different type of phosphate binders is different and they should be taken with your meal or just before. Check with your dietitian when you need to take them.

Eating a low-phosphate diet is not as straightforward as it sounds. It is very difficult to cut down phosphate intake without also eating less protein.

Patients who need to adjust their diet to reduce their blood phosphate level will be given specific advice by their dietitian. This will probably include asking them to be careful about eating dairy products (eggs, milk, cheese, yoghurt), offal (liver, kidneys, heart) and shellfish – as these all contain very high amounts of phosphate. The dietitian may also give advice about when and how to take the phosphate-binding tablets.

In general, patients only need to worry about the amount of phosphate in their diet if their doctor or dietitian specifically tells them they have a problem.

Potassium

Potassium is very important mineral in the human body. Healthy kidneys control the potassium level without any difficulty, but in kidney failure this doesn't happen. Potassium levels may then be either too high or too low (see the reference section for more detail).

The main problem with potassium is that if it rises too high or falls too low, it becomes dangerous to the heart, affecting the electrical activity of the heart and can lead to the heart stopping. So it is very important to keep the potassium at safe levels.

Potassium is one of the substances that is measured when dialysis patients have blood tests. Any patient who regularly has high blood potassium levels will be seen by the dietitian often. The dietitian will try to find out if the person is eating anything that might be causing a high level of potassium in the blood.

Many foods contain potassium, but some have more than others. Kidney patients whose blood potassium levels are high or rising will normally be asked to restrict their intake of high-potassium foods. This will involve avoiding some foods, such as chocolate and crisps, and eating less of other potassium containing foods, such as bananas, oranges and mushrooms. If this dietary restriction does not work, there may be a need to have more dialysis (if that has been started) by spending longer on the dialysis machine or doing extra exchanges of PD.

However, patients on more frequent or continuous forms of dialysis such as daily home haemodialysis, night-time haemodialysis, or PD rarely need to restrict their potassium intake. In fact, they may sometimes need to increase it. This is because more frequent dialysis generally clears potassium from the blood very effectively.

Hospital or satellite-based haemodialysis, on the other hand, is an intermittent process. So, in the intervals between dialysis, the blood potassium may begin to rise. These patients may therefore need dietary advice on potassium intake.

Unless their doctor or dietitian tells them otherwise, kidney patients can assume that they do not have a problem with their blood potassium.

What about salt and fluid?

Salt and fluid advice is often given together. A salty diet may make patients thirsty, and make life very uncomfortable if you have been asked to limit the amount of fluid you drink.

Salt restriction usually involves the following:

- using little or no salt in cooking and at the table (don't use 'low salt' replacements as they contain potassium);

- eating very few high-salt foods (these are mainly convenience and processed foods).

Hospital or satellite-based haemodialysis patients often have greater restrictions on fluid intake as their dialysis is intermittent and fluid can build up in between sessions. They therefore need to be extra careful about the amount of salt they eat.

Advice about how much you can safely drink is based on how much urine is passed (if you still pass urine) and the amount of water removed by dialysis. Generally speaking, the more urine patients pass, the more fluid they can drink. Most dialysis patients can drink 500 ml of fluid every day plus the equivalent of any urine they have passed plus any fluid lost by dialysis on the previous day. For many patients, this works out to be about 1 litre a day for in-centre haemodialysis patients and 1.5 litres for PD patients. Many people who do more frequent haemodialysis at home can often drink more. This is because they can remove fluid every time they have dialysis, which can be six or seven times a week.

Vitamin supplements

Most doctors and dietitians agree that the fat-soluble vitamins (i.e. vitamins A, D, E and K) are rarely a problem for people with kidney failure and therefore don't need to be taken as supplements. Supplements of fat-soluble vitamins may even cause problems, as they can mount up in the body.

One fat-soluble vitamin – vitamin A (found in large amounts in cod and halibut liver oil capsules) – is known to be toxic and can cause particular problems if taken to excess.

Water-soluble vitamins (i.e. vitamins B and C) are lost during dialysis (both PD and HD). It is therefore possible that dialysis patients may need to take supplements. This might be more important if they have had to eat less of some foods because of potassium restrictions.

Diet before starting dialysis

People with kidney failure who have not yet started dialysis should follow normal healthy eating guidelines.

This includes continuing to eat foods that contain protein even after the level of urea in their blood has started to rise.

If people with kidney failure restrict their intake of dietary protein, their urea level will not rise so quickly. For this reason, in the past, patients were asked to reduce the amount of protein in the diet which could delay the need for dialysis. However, restricting protein is controversial, since this can lead to malnutrition – i.e. they do not get enough protein to keep healthy. However, in some countries (e.g. Italy) doctors still recommend reducing protein intake, by use of a vegetarian diet.

When the time for dialysis draws closer, some people do not feel as hungry as they used to – and some foods, particularly meat products, may taste 'funny'. Special dietary supplements may help such patients to maintain adequate protein, energy and vitamin intakes. A dietitian will be able to provide advice about these supplements.

Diet during dialysis

Diet is very important for patients on dialysis. All kidney patients are at risk of developing malnutrition so it is important to eat properly.

It may also be necessary to pay special attention to a dialysis patient's intake of phosphate, calcium, potassium, salt, fluid and vitamins. Most people having dialysis will also have to control the amount of fluid they drink to prevent fluid overload.

Gaining weight and kidney failure

Weight gain (obesity) can be an issue for people with kidney failure.

Obesity can actually be one of the causes of kidney failure. This is because being overweight makes a person much more likely to develop diabetes, one of the major causes of kidney failure. Obesity itself is a recognised cause of kidney failure without diabetes being present.

Reversing obesity (losing weight by dieting) will not cure kidney failure. However, being a healthy weight has lots of other health advantages, such as reducing blood pressure and strain on the heart.

Patients on the transplant waiting list are more likely to cope physically with a transplant operation if they are a healthy weight and do not have raised blood pressure.

Obesity can cause practical problems for people on dialysis. Overweight people with fat arms can have particular problems with access for haemodialysis. Their veins can be difficult to reach, or weak, and therefore difficult to make a fistula from. It can be difficult to put a PD catheter into someone who has a very fat abdomen. Very obese patients will be too unfit to be offered a transplant.

If obesity is a problem, healthy eating guidelines may help. Overweight patients should ask to be referred to a dietitian for advice.

Losing weight and kidney failure

Some kidney patients find they lose a lot of weight and become very thin. This is usually because they are not eating enough (especially foods providing protein and energy). Loss of appetite is often one of the first things people notice when their kidneys stop working properly.

This can lead to malnutrition. So, to prevent malnutrition, some patients on dialysis will be asked to increase their food intake – especially their intake of protein.

The main cause of malnutrition in kidney patients is probably the simplest one – poor appetite. This is one of the major symptoms of kidney failure, and is often the reason why people go to their family doctor in the first place.

When someone is pre-dialysis (or has a failing

transplant), worsening of the appetite is one of the reasons why doctors start (or restart) dialysis. When a patient is on dialysis, a change – hopefully an improvement – in their appetite is often the most reliable guide to the effectiveness of the dialysis. It can tell more than any of the blood tests.

Dialysis usually returns a kidney patient's appetite to near normal, although few dialysis patients ever really have a 'good' appetite.

If a patient is not receiving enough dialysis, loss of appetite is one of the first symptoms to return. An increase in the dialysis may then help to improve the patient's appetite. However, only a transplant will fully return a patient to a 'normal' appetite.

A build-up of toxins in the blood may not be the only reason for appetite problems in a kidney patient. Severe anaemia may also lead to a poor appetite.

Also, PD patients may have a poor appetite because of the dialysis fluid in their abdomen, which can make them feel bloated.

Other causes of weight loss

In addition to appetite problems, a number of other factors may contribute to the increased risk of weight loss in kidney patients on dialysis.

PD patients lose protein and amino acids (substances from which proteins are built up) into their bags of dialysis fluid. Haemodialysis patients also lose amino acids into their dialysis fluid. So kidney patients on both types of dialysis need extra protein in their diet to make up for these losses.

Poor control of blood acidity level (blood tends to be acidic in kidney failure) is another reason that people with kidney failure become malnourished. Acidity is shown by the bicarbonate levels in the blood.

Infections also increase a person's requirements for high-protein and high-energy foods, and infections tend to be more common in dialysis patients.

A further possible cause of malnutrition in kidney patients may be that some patients are not eating enough because of dietary restrictions imposed by their doctor or dietitian.

Loss of weight tends to be more common in haemodialysis than PD patients. PD patients have an extra source of calories – the sugar contained in PD fluid. Some of this is absorbed by the patient, providing the equivalent of approximately 300–500 calories a day – similar to eating between one and two Mars bars. Haemodialysis patients don't have this extra energy source and may need to eat more and perhaps take supplements.

Individual dietary recommendations

All people with kidney failure are advised, as far as possible, to follow 'healthy eating guidelines' (i.e. to eat a high-fibre, moderate-fat and low-salt diet). But in some cases, specific individual priorities will over-ride these guidelines.

The most common example of going against the usual guidelines is if someone is losing a lot of weight and needs to boost their intake of calories by eating more fatty food. In this situation, malnutrition is a more serious and immediate danger than any possible future increased risk of heart disease from a high-fat diet.

Diet after a transplant

If a kidney transplant is functioning well, then there is no need to be on a special diet. If the transplant starts to fail, the situation may be different.

Transplant patients, being immunosuppressed and at greater risk of picking up infections, should be given information about food hygiene. In addition, they will be advised to follow normal healthy eating guidelines. This is particularly important because of two problems associated with a transplant. These problems are:
- excessive weight gain (usually a side effect of taking steroid drugs, such as prednisolone); and
- high cholesterol levels.

Both of these problems increase the risk of heart disease. Healthy eating along with regular exercise may help reduce the risk.

Taking control of what you eat

Diet is an area where you really can take some control over your life and feel you are doing something to improve your own situation. Having kidney failure does not mean you have to stop enjoying your food. What it does mean is that you need to understand what you are eating, and learn which foods you can eat as much of as you like; which foods you should have once in a while (as a treat) and which foods you really should consider cutting out altogether. It is important, though, that while you follow your doctor and dietitian's advice, you do not become so obsessed with watching everything you eat that meals become a chore for you.

The Further Reading section lists some books that will help you find the right balance.

Being active and exercising

People who are not active and don't take regular exercise are at a high risk of getting heart disease, having a stroke, developing diabetes, cancer and dementia. Being inactive can also lead to depression.

So, just as for everyone else, it's important that people with kidney failure are active.

However, people with kidney failure may not feel as strong as they used to; they may also feel tired and weak, which can make it difficult to be active.

There are three main reasons why this happens:

- wastes build up in the body because the kidneys cannot get rid of them;
- many people with kidney failure also have anaemia which causes tiredness and breathlessness;
- excess wastes in the blood and anaemia can make patients feel too poorly to do much. This then means that they lose fitness and strength, and feel even more tired.

Benefits of physical activity for kidney patients

Keeping fit has many health benefits. For people with kidney failure these include;

- improving your quality of life;
- improving the quality of your sleep;
- improving general well-being and mood;
- building up muscles;
- preventing weight gain or losing weight;
- protecting the heart from disease and making it stronger;
- helping to control blood pressure;
- helping to reduce cholesterol levels in the blood;
- helping to control diabetes if you have it and prevent it if you don't;
- helping to make your bones stronger.

Exercise advice

All of us should try to get about 30 minutes of exercise on at least 4 days a week. This should be at a level that makes you get a little out of breath.

If you haven't done any exercise for a while, you may need to build this up gradually. Also, you don't need to do the 30 minutes all in one go. For example you may go for a brisk walk for 15 minutes twice a day. It's important to take a rest if you need to.

You won't make much difference to your fitness if you only exercise once or twice each week.

Building muscle strength is also important and so you should try to include some strength exercises about twice a week.

Moderate physical activity is good for most people but you should always check with your doctor or other members of your health care team before you start an exercise regime. This is particularly important if you have another health problem such as diabetes, heart or liver disease. Your doctor or nurse can tell what exercise is best for you because they know about your condition and treatment and what you can and can't do.

It is fine to exercise to a point where you feel tired and a bit short of breath and your muscles ache afterwards.

However, you should not exercise to the point of exhaustion and you shouldn't exercise if you are feeling unwell. If you start to feel unwell during exercise you should stop immediately, particularly if you feel:

- unusually weak or breathless;
- dizzy or nauseous;
- pain.

It is best not to exercise on a full stomach, and people on peritoneal dialysis (PD) may find it easier to exercise with an empty abdomen rather than one filled with PD fluid.

For people on dialysis who have either an arteriovenous (AV) fistula in their arm for haemodialysis or an abdominal catheter for PD, lifting weights should be discussed with your doctor first. Your doctor may recommend that you lift light weights to avoid harm to your vascular access. Lifting even light weights every other day can help increase blood flow, build muscle and help you become stronger. Lifting weights can be done while watching television in your home or at your local gym in a weight room. You should always check with your doctors or dialysis nurse to find out if there are any special precautions you need to take so you do not harm your fistula.

Exercise can take many forms – from the sporty challenges of playing team sports such as football, rugby or netball, to the more gentle activities such as bowling, gardening, walking or yoga.

Doing even a small amount of physical exercise – such as housework or reorganising the furniture in a room – is good. Once you start to feel the benefits, you will be motivated to carry on and your fitness, in turn, will continue to improve.

KEY FACTS

1 Advice about what you should eat will vary according to the stage of kidney failure and the type of treatment you are receiving.

2 'Healthy eating guidelines' – for a high-fibre, moderate-fat and low-salt diet – are generally recommended whether you are waiting for dialysis, are on dialysis or have a transplant.

3 It is difficult to measure someone's nutritional state. The blood albumin level is often used, but is not very reliable. A low level may be a sign of malnutrition in some cases.

4 You should only alter your diet when your kidney doctor or dietitian advises you to.

5 Weight gain can lead to practical problems if you need dialysis. It may also make you too unfit for a transplant operation.

6 Weight loss and malnutrition are the major problems for many patients on dialysis. So, for these patients, eating a lot of high-protein food may be recommended.

7 If you are on frequent or continuous dialysis treatments such as PD or daily home haemodialysis, it is unlikely you will need to reduce your potassium intake. But you may need to restrict it if you are on hospital or satellite-based haemodialysis three times a week.

8 Eating a lot of salt or salty foods will make you thirsty. You may need to restrict your salt intake, particularly if fluid is restricted.

9 If you have had a transplant, you are unlikely to have any dietary restrictions. But you should try to follow standard healthy eating guidelines.

KEY FACTS *continued*

10 Taking regular exercise is important for everyone, especially people with kidney failure. It has many advantages for your health and wellbeing.

11 You should exercise for at least 30 minutes 4 or 5 times a week.

12 Any form of physical exercise is good, and the more you do, the better you will feel.

9 LIVING LIFE TO THE FULL

This chapter looks at the reasons why people with kidney failure may feel differently from people with healthy kidneys. It also suggests ways of coping with the psychological problems you may experience. The chapter also looks at adapting to life with kidney failure, going back to work and travelling.

Introduction

Being told that you have kidney failure has a massive impact. It will affect the whole of your life, not just your physical condition. Once you know you have kidney failure, you will have to make changes to the way you live. You are also likely to find the illness affects the way you feel about yourself, and your priorities in life. Kidney failure may also affect those around you including your family, friends and even your work colleagues.

Body and mind

Everyone's psychological and emotional well-being has a major impact on their physical well-being. The way you feel will influence the way you behave. If you have kidney failure, the way that you behave can have a direct effect on your health. For example, you may become less careful about your diet, forget to take your tablets, or abandon fluid restrictions – all of which put additional strain on an already poorly body.

Psychological needs

Psychology is about behaviour: why people behave the way they do, and how they can change the way they behave. It is about how people feel about themselves, their situation, the people who are part of their lives.

Everybody has psychological needs – not just people who happen to have kidney failure. However old or ill we might be, we all need to be heard, understood and valued. Illness can make this more difficult. People who are unwell may find it hard to express their fears and anxieties and may feel out of control of their situation.

Stresses on people with kidney failure

Any long-term or life-threatening illness can be extremely stressful. Any change – even a pleasant change like getting married – is stressful. When changes are 'negative', however, stress will be greatly increased.

The treatment of kidney failure means you can't avoid changes in lifestyle. People have to adapt their usual routine. They may have to make changes to their eating and drinking habits. They may not have enough energy to continue working or to pursue their hobbies or interests.

Some of the stresses that commonly affect people with kidney failure are:

- having to make decisions about things they have never even thought about before;

- taking in strange information, to enable them to understand a complex medical subject;
- learning about themselves and the ways they cope with things;
- needing to ask for support to manage their treatment;
- seeing themselves as a complete person, not just as a disease or condition;
- learning to live differently for the rest of their life; and
- worrying about the future.

Changes to the expected progression of life may also cause stress. For example, it may be difficult for a young person to leave home, either because they have kidney failure, or because they feel they should look after a parent with kidney failure. Sometimes people have to cope with unpleasant reactions from their employers and work colleagues. Later in life, retirement may come early and be totally unwelcome.

Other members of the family also have to make adjustments. Kidney failure has an impact on their lives too. The normal pattern of life is disrupted and relationships have to be redefined.

The diagnosis

For some people, the diagnosis of kidney failure comes completely out of the blue. This can be extremely difficult to cope with. Even when kidney failure was already suspected, knowing it is certain can cause difficulties. The way that the diagnosis is given, and the quality of support offered immediately afterwards, can make a big difference to a person's future well-being.

Initial reactions

Following a diagnosis of kidney failure (or any other serious long-term illness), people often go through the following stages:

1 **Shock.** At first, patients (and often also family members and friends) go into a state of shock, feeling stunned, bewildered or strangely detached – as though they are observing life rather than being part of it. This shock can last a short while or may continue for weeks.

2 **Grief.** Then people begin to react to the news, often with feelings of loss, grief, helplessness and despair. They may feel overwhelmed by reality, and find it difficult to think clearly or plan effectively.

3 **Denial.** One very common reaction to serious illness is to deny the existence of the disease or its implications. But the problem does not go away, the symptoms get worse, and there are reminders from other people that the illness exists.

4 **Acceptance.** Gradually, people come to accept reality a little at a time, and begin to make progress towards adapting successfully to their condition.

Longer-term problems

Patients with kidney failure often experience longer-term psychological problems too. Some of these are described below:

1 **Lack of co-operation with the healthcare team.** As described in Chapter 2 the long-term care for kidney patients is a partnership approach between the healthcare professionals, patients and their loved ones. This partnership is based on cooperation and understanding from everyone involved.

Occasionally, particularly if a patient feels stressed, depressed or overwhelmed by the situation, it can lead to them becoming withdrawn and un-cooperative. In some situations this can lead to the patient not keeping to the decisions that have been agreed for their treatment and lifestyle. This can be because:

- they believe that the treatment is not effective, and there is no obvious benefit from it;
- they do not know what effect the treatment is supposed to have, or why it is important to continue with it; and
- the side effects of the treatment are unpleasant.

Many patients will have at least one period when they find it difficult to follow the guidance set out by their doctors and nurses. It's important to seek help, and to talk about how you feel if this happens to you, as there may be very serious risks to your health.

There may be ways that you can have some flexibility with your treatments. However, it is always important to be absolutely certain that changing your treatment plan is not life-treatening. Please talk to your renal team first.

If you understand why you should (or should not) be doing something, you will feel much more motivated to do it.

2 **Anxiety.** As well as the anxieties felt by most people at some time in their lives, kidney patients have additional anxieties relating to their condition and its treatment. Some possible problem areas include:

- relationships (e.g. 'We can't share the same interests any more'; 'We've both changed so much');
- quality of life (e.g. 'I miss walking the dog'; 'I'd planned to go abroad');
- employment (e.g. 'I've taken too much time off work');
- practical management (e.g. 'How can I do my dialysis myself when I feel so ill?'); and
- understanding (e.g. 'I can't understand all the medical words').

3 **Body image.** Some people who have kidney failure experience problems with their changed body image. They may see their fistula or PD catheter as a fault in their body. They feel horribly scarred and find it really hard to look at themselves.

The perceptions of patients and medical staff can differ widely here. When doctors and nurses talk about a 'really good fistula', they are talking about the ease of access, the rate of blood flow, and the strength of the blood vessels. What the patient experiences is a forearm with a continuous buzzing sensation, and a disfiguring swelling where it used to be smooth and flat. Some patients cannot see their fistula as a 'good' thing at all.

4 **Awareness of the end of life.** People with kidney failure know that without treatment they would die. Having to live with this sort of knowledge puts a very different perspective on life's priorities.

5 **Dependency and self-confidence.** Many people with kidney failure feel that they are very dependent on others; on hospital doctors and nurses, and on their partners, relatives and friends. People with kidney failure have to deal with the fact that their life depends on a machine, on PD bags, or on someone else's kidney. This can weaken a person's confidence in coping with many aspects of life.

Talking to your healthcare team, a counsellor or a friend or relative can really help to put things in perspective. You can ask to see a psychologist if your renal unit has one. Other places where you can get support are charities and support groups. See Useful Addresses and Websites for a list of where to get help.

6 **Sense of loss.** A healthy person will take their body (including their kidneys) for granted, never having to think about them. Sometimes the failure of this essential body part can cause a sense of loss or grieving.

7 **Depression.** Many people get depressed at some stage in their lives. People with kidney failure are no exception. There are times when they feel low, and to do anything at all requires a huge effort; times when they should allow themselves to feel sorry for themselves; and times to cry.

8 **Changes to treatment.** One of the many difficult things about kidney failure is that the treatment changes over time. For example, patients may change from PD to haemodialysis, or vice versa, or they may receive a transplant, or resume dialysis after a transplant fails.

Change can be stressful, even it if is seen to be a positive change such as having a transplant. Having got into a routine, and feeling settled, it can be disturbing to have normality disrupted.

9 **Ageing and bereavement.** It is not only a patient's treatment that changes. Everyone changes to some extent as they get older. Tasks that seem easy when someone is young may become more troublesome as the years go by. Coping with kidney failure may become more difficult.

Everyone – especially those in perfect health – finds that, as they get older, more and more of their friends will die. This can be a particular problem for older patients in the kidney unit. In addition, if you attend the same unit for a long time, you may see many staff changes. Just as you are building up a rapport with one dialysis nurse, they move to a new job or retire. This can become a strong and supportive relationship and the better it is, the more difficult you may find it to adjust to their not being around.

10 **Sexual activity.** Sexual problems are common among people with kidney failure and can put a strain on a relationship. There may be a loss of sex drive. For many young men, the most distressing aspect of kidney failure is their inability to get or maintain a normal erection. Your GP or a specialist may be able to help with this problem.

It is a good idea to talk about problems with your partner if they arise. It may even be helpful to seek professional advice from a sex counsellor or from an organisation such as Relate.

11 **Conflicting advice.** People with kidney failure receive information from lots of different people. The people who pass on this information have themselves already interpreted it according to their own backgrounds and beliefs. So, what a patient hears may not always be totally true. The advice from one source may be different to advice from another. It is not surprising that kidney patients are sometimes confused by what they are told.

If you find yourself in a situation where you are being told different things by different people in your healthcare team, it is important to speak up and say that you are confused. Sometimes, there are different opinions amongst healthcare professionals and there is not always a wrong or a right answer. Talking about the options can help to make more sense of the situation.

12 **Poor concentration.** Patients sometimes worry that kidney failure may be affecting their brain. They may find that they sometimes cannot concentrate as well, or think as clearly, as they used to before their kidneys failed. This can be caused by a build-up of the wastes in your blood and may be improved by dialysis treatment or a transplant.

If you suffer from poor concentration, speak to your doctor or nurse at the renal unit.

Factors affecting the ability to cope

Some people cope more easily than others with the psychological and emotional aspects of kidney failure.

A person's ability to cope with illness is affected by a range of things:

1 **Illness-related factors**
   - Some people are more afraid than others of the possible consequences of kidney failure. Fears of disability, deformity, pain or early death can cause problems. The more a person feels threatened by their illness, the harder they will find it to cope.
   - Kidney failure often occurs together with other conditions, such as diabetes, anaemia and renal bone disease. These conditions cause their own symptoms, giving kidney patients even more things to worry about.
   - Some people have to cope with unpleasant side effects from the tablets they must take (particularly if they have had a transplant, see Chapter 6).
   - The treatment of kidney failure involves major time commitments, which can interfere with finding or holding down a job. Lack of secure employment can be an additional strain.
   - Kidney failure requires patients and their families to make changes in their lifestyle. These

changes may put pressure on relationships and increase stress.

- Many people with a chronic illness, such as kidney failure, feel self-conscious about their disease and want to hide it from others. This can cause stress and make it harder to cope.

2 **Age.** The age at which a person develops kidney failure is likely to have an effect on the way they will cope:

- Children may not understand the long-term implications of the condition.
- Adolescents need to be liked and accepted by their peers. Because of this, some may neglect their medical care to avoid appearing different from their friends.
- Young adults with kidney failure may feel they no longer have the chance to develop their lives in the direction they planned – to get married, to have children, or to enter a particular career. Such feelings may cause anger and resentment.
- Middle-aged patients may have problems adjusting to the disruption of an established lifestyle. They may find themselves unable to finish tasks they have started, such as building up a career.
- Older patients may resent not being able to enjoy their retirement in the way they had planned.

3 **Personality.** Aspects of a person's personality can affect their ability to cope with kidney failure.

- People who cope well with long-term health problems tend to have hardy or resilient personalities which allow them to see good in difficult situations. They are able to balance hope against despair and to find purpose in life whatever happens. They maintain their self-esteem and resist feeling helpless and hopeless.
- Kidney failure often means that patients must take on a dependent and passive role, for a while at least. Some people find this especially difficult since it is so different from the independent role they have developed over the years.

4 **Social and cultural factors.** A person's ability to cope with illness is also affected by their background.

- People from different social, cultural and religious backgrounds will have different ways of dealing with situations. Problems may arise if doctors and nurses fail to take this into account.
- People's beliefs about health come from a number of sources, including the media, advertising, other patients' experiences and their friends. These beliefs may be incorrect or only half true.
- Sometimes, misconceptions can add to the difficulties of adjusting to kidney failure. For instance, people who believe that nothing is seriously wrong unless they are in pain are not likely to seek help for a condition that has no obvious symptoms, such as high blood pressure.

5 **Support.** The amount and quality of support available to patients are further influences on how well they cope with kidney failure.

- People who live alone, away from their family and with few friends, tend to adjust poorly to long-term diseases. Other forms of support are particularly important for these people.
- For many people with kidney failure, their immediate family is the main source of psychological support. For others, this role is taken by one or more close friends. Such support is usually a big help to the person. However, it is also true that relatives and friends sometimes undermine effective coping by providing bad examples or poor advice.
- Hospitals do not always provide people with kidney failure with the support they need. Unfortunately, at present, not all renal units have a clinical psychologist. However, there is a general recognition of the need to provide

patients with psychological support, and some nurses have had special training in counselling.

- For some people, lack of practical support at home may be a problem. Patients may have difficulty getting round the house or doing everyday tasks. Many lack equipment that could help them become more self-sufficient.
- Many support groups have been set up by and for people with kidney failure. These groups can provide emotional and sometimes financial support, as well as information. (See Useful Addresses and Websites for more ideas of where to get help and support).

Coping strategies

People use different strategies to help them cope with long-term illness. Many kidney patients find the following strategies helpful:

1 **Denial.** In the early stages, it can be very useful to deny the situation or not to take it seriously. This helps people escape from the feeling of being overwhelmed by the disease. It also allows time to organise other, better ways of dealing with the situation.

2 **Information seeking.** People often find it helpful to seek information about their disease and its treatment. Becoming expert in a subject may give you a sense of control over it. It is particularly important that you feel able to ask your doctor or nurse questions, and that you ask them to explain anything they have told you in words that are easy for you to understand. There is also a great deal of other information available, from books and websites. The quality of this information does vary considerably, but all the sources listed in Useful Addresses and Websites have been looked at by the authors and have been found to be reliable.

3 **Disease management.** Many patients gain a sense of control over their disease by becoming involved in its management – including being responsible for taking medicines and doing their own dialysis at home.

Some people find it helpful to keep their own records (for example, of their blood pressure, creatinine, eGFR, Hb, potassium and phosphate levels). Patient View is an excellent way to manage the information about your care. You may also wish to keep a record of what was said during appointments at the renal clinic (dated, and with a record of which doctors, nurses, dieticians and other professionals were seen and what decisions were made); details and dates of any operations or other procedures undergone, together with the names of the surgeon, anaesthetist and any other health professionals involved.

4 **Goal setting.** A very useful coping strategy for many people is to set themselves appropriate goals. These might include, for example, exercising or going out, getting back to work and trying to maintain regular routines. It may be that you have a big event you'd like to attend such as a wedding or a special holiday.

5 **Prioritising different activities.** Some people with kidney failure find it can be helpful in the long term to reduce the importance of some of their current activities, such as social drinking or playing contact sports. Maintaining some of the things you did before you had kidney failure is also important. Work, education and travel may have been a significant part of life, and with planning, are perfectly possible to continue.

Working

Most employers are very accommodating towards people with kidney failure. Keeping them informed of changes to your treatment and the frequency of hospital visits help with their understanding of your requirements.

People who have their dialysis at home often don't have a problem fitting work into their life. Home dialysis (either PD or haemodialysis) is flexible and, if dialysis is done overnight (by APD for example), it may interfere very little with work schedules. Hospital or satellite-based haemodialysis may be more difficult to fit into a job. However, the renal unit may be able to offer a 'dialysis slot' that enables work to continue.

People who have a successful kidney transplant are usually able to work. However, in the early days after the operation, visits to the hospital can be much more frequent, especially if the patient was on a home-based treatment before the transplant where hospital visits are infrequent. It's important to keep employers informed so they are prepared for possible disruptions to work patterns.

Travel and holidays

One of the ways in which kidney patients can enjoy full and productive lives is by taking a holiday or business trip. For many people with kidney failure, travel to most parts of the world is perfectly possible; however, planning is essential. Last-minute bookings are not a realistic option. There is plenty of help available with the planning process, beginning with your renal unit. Travel can give close family members a welcome break too.

Staff at the renal unit can help you decide if you are ready to travel. They can advise you on suitable destinations according to the treatment you are on. They can help you make appointments in other renal units so you can be monitored or treated while travelling.

Before planning anything, talk to your renal unit.

Anyone with a pre-existing medical condition will need a letter from a doctor confirming that they are fit to travel in order to get travel insurance. This includes transplant patients. For more information about travel and holidays, visit the websites recommended in the back of this book or contact the Kidney Care UK. Your doctor or renal care team can also provide you with information about any immunisations required.

Short trips away are possible for patients on dialysis. Those on haemodialysis can plan a short trip away between dialysis sessions – especially on the two-day gap (e.g. Saturday and Sunday or Sunday and Monday).

Peritoneal dialysis patients, on the other hand, are free to travel any time as supplies can be taken along in the car. For longer trips away, PD supplies can be delivered to most parts of the world and will be waiting for you when you arrive at your destination. It's even possible to have PD on a cruise, or while camping.

Haemodialysis patients wishing to take a longer break away from home will need to organise dialysis in a unit near to their destination. Holiday dialysis centres are available in many parts of the world but need to be booked in advance.

KEY FACTS

1 Kidney failure has a major impact on the whole of a patient's life.

2 People with kidney failure have to cope with extra stresses.

3 Kidney failure and its treatment will affect the lives of those who are closest to you, as well as your own.

4 People diagnosed with kidney failure usually go through shock, grief and denial before acceptance.

5 Not keeping to the treatment guidance that you have been given can be very dangerous and even cause death – so it is vital you ask your doctor to talk through any aspect of your treatment programme you don't feel happy with or find difficult.

6 Other long-term problems may include anxiety, problems with body image, loss of self-confidence, depression, adapting to changes, and a loss of interest in sex.

7 Kidney failure can sometimes affect a person's ability to concentrate and think clearly.

8 Many factors affect a person's ability to cope with kidney failure, but there are various coping strategies that different people find useful.

9 Some people prefer not to think about the situation (denial). Others may adopt a structured approach, managing their own illness as far as possible, doing their dialysis at home, prioritising different activities or goal setting. It is important you follow the approach that works best for you.

10 Maintaining some of the things you did before you had kidney failure is important. It is perfectly possible to continue work, education and travel but they may require advance planning.

10 END OF LIFE CARE

This chapter explores some of those difficult issues around the subject of death and dying. The intention is to give readers the information necessary to make choices at the appropriate time – the best choices for them and those they love. We also discuss what happens if you choose not to have any treatment for kidney failure, either dialysis or a transplant.

Introduction

Death is a subject that isn't always discussed openly with patients in a dialysis unit. Dialysis and kidney transplants are successful in treating an otherwise fatal illness. These treatments are all about life. Yet nobody can attend a kidney unit without realising that death is always a possibility for them. In a large dialysis centre, a week rarely passes without someone dying.

Renal units are close communities, where patients often know each other as friends. When there is a death at the unit most of the patients will be aware and this can remind them of their own mortality.

People with kidney failure live with the knowledge that they have a shorter life expectancy than the rest of the population. Their cause of death is not usually directly because of kidney failure. The most common cause of death in people on dialysis is heart and other cardiovascular diseases. Another common cause of death is through serious infection.

Do I have to have dialysis?

Some people opt to stop dialysis treatment or decide that they don't want to have dialysis treatment at all. Without replacing kidney function when it is reduced to a very low level means that a person will die of their kidney failure. These difficult choices reflect the fact that dialysis can be a burden for some people and may neither extend nor improve life.

There is no doubt that life on dialysis can be full, rewarding and worthwhile for many people. However, there are some who feel either that they would not wish to live with the restrictions and problems of treatment, or that they have done so for long enough. For people with a lot of other long-term medical problems dialysis may not prolong life. So, when anyone is thinking about dialysis in particular, it is about weighing up the benefits – potentially a prolonged or improved life – against the down side – the burden of the treatment itself.

For example, frail and elderly patients who are having haemodialysis in the hospital or a satellite unit often need hospital transport to get them to and from their dialysis sessions. This can be exhausting and may mean that other aspects of their life are affected. They may be unsteady after a session and just need to go to bed. They may need to leave home very early in the morning or they may arrive home very late at night. This can impact on sleep patterns. The dialysis sessions may also interfere with mealtimes and many patients just don't get the chance to eat on

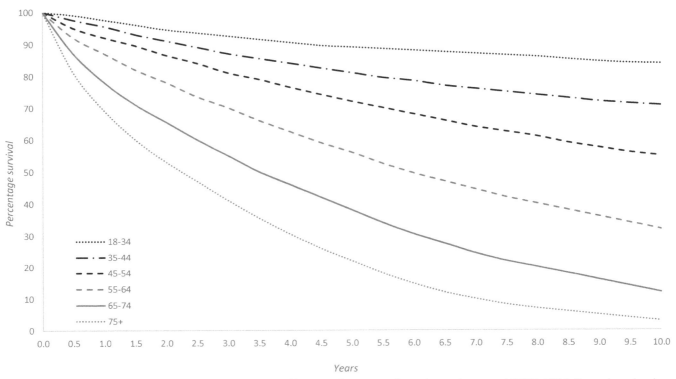

Figure 10.1: Survival of kidney patients in years, grouped by age. Statistics collected over the period 1997–2015. Reproduced with permission from the UK Renal Registry 20th Annual Report

dialysis days. This can have a big impact on energy levels, nutrition and general health. So, for haemodialysis, the treatment is not just the hours on the machine. It is the getting to and from the unit, the treatment itself and the time it takes to get back to your best – the recovery time.

Some aspects of this can be tackled with a bit of 'lateral thinking'. Having dialysis at home can be an option, if the right support is available. It gets rid of the travel aspects and there is no waiting around. Both PD and home HD carried out more frequently – but for fewer hours – reduces the recovery time for many. Some people may need support but a relative or carer may be able to help with the dialysis. This is more often the case for people

who have PD, but patients on home HD often have support from a relative. In some cases, a paid and trained carer may help. Assisted PD has become a practical option and has helped many people to live at home, even at the end of their life.

It is important for patients and their families to understand that dialysis is not compulsory. If you do not wish to receive treatment, or decide that you wish to stop dialysis, you should discuss this with the staff at your renal unit. If the kidneys have failed, not having dialysis treatment will mean that the patient will die, usually within a few days or weeks, depending on their degree of kidney failure. Just remember, we are talking about making choices for the future.

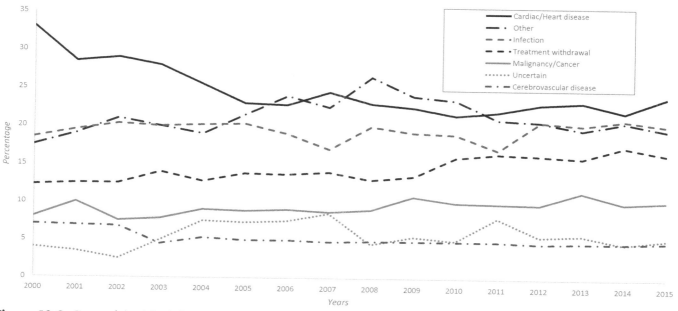

Figure 10.2: Cause of death for kidney patients over the period 2000–2015. Reproduced with permission from the UK Renal Registry 20th Annual Report

Patients and their families are the only people who can judge whether quality of life with dialysis is acceptable for them, but the team as a whole are there to offer their expertise and advice – to support and share in this important decision. You may be frail or elderly, severely disabled or restricted, yet satisfied that life is still worthwhile.

Deciding not to have dialysis or to stop having dialysis are big decisions and the team is there to help you. Let us talk about these options in more detail.

The decision not to start dialysis treatment (also known as conservative care)

Some patients decide that they do not want any dialysis at all. This choice is often called 'conservative care'. It is a choice made by some patients, supported by their family and clinical team, when they think dialysis will not help.

If a person attending a pre-dialysis clinic tells the consultant that, when the need arises, he or she does not want dialysis treatment, it is important that this decision is made with full knowledge – it is an 'informed' choice. It is also important to know that it is acceptable to change the decision later.

In the first place, the patient needs to ask the doctor, quite directly, about the outcome, i.e. how long they might expect to live both with and without dialysis, and what can be done to make their last days comfortable if they choose not to dialyse. This information is essential for making a rational decision.

It may be that, with a special diet and medication, a person would live for some months, free of frequent hospital visits or preparation for treatment such as access surgery for a fistula or PD catheter. This is particularly true in the case of very elderly people, who are leading an inactive life.

It is important to be aware that it is impossible to know exactly what life on dialysis is like unless one has experienced it. Even talking to others receiving treatment does not give the full picture, as everyone is different. Sometimes, patients agree to treatment reluctantly, only to find that it is not as bad as they had imagined it would be. Others tell us that, on the contrary, they had expected it to be much easier to cope with, or that they had hoped to feel far better on treatment than they actually do.

Having dialysis will prolong life in most (but not all) people, so weighing up the risks and benefits of not having treatment is very important for each individual.

Trials of dialysis

To discover what life on dialysis is like, some patients opt for a 'trial of dialysis', lasting a few weeks or months. This allows them to discover both the good and bad sides of life on dialysis, and to decide whether the benefits outweigh the drawbacks. In some cases, a short period of treatment may be undertaken in order to give patients time to settle their affairs or resolve conflicting feelings in the family.

Others need time to allow visits from family members living abroad, and to say goodbye. Everything should be done that will allow the patient peace of mind. Relatives, too, need a sense of resolution, free from unnecessary guilt and regret.

The decision to stop dialysis

Some people who have been on dialysis for a long time and are elderly or have lots of other health problems may wish to stop dialysis.

Nobody can force a patient to attend for dialysis. Sometimes, the very knowledge that they are able to stop when they wish is enough to give individuals the will to carry on for the present.

Patients sometimes fear that they are 'letting down' the staff of the kidney unit by wanting to stop treatment.

It can seem like ingratitude, or a rejection of the care they have been given. While staff will be sad, they may also be relieved, having been aware of the person's distress. They should, in any case, respect the patient's decision. Nobody can know fully what life is like for another person.

There are many reasons why a decision to stop dialysis may be taken. The most common reason is that the patient suffers a medical setback, often unrelated to the kidneys, such as a stroke or, for example, a patient with diabetes who needs to have a limb amputated. Another serious health problem would result in further disability and limitation, which the patient might regard as just too much to cope with. Life on dialysis may have been tolerable, but the additional problem may remove what quality remained in the patient's life. Loss of independence is often the deciding factor.

The second most common reason for withdrawal is the gradual deterioration caused by ageing and the complications of many years of dialysis. The patient may have considerable pain and restriction from renal bone disease, or problems with blood circulation from narrowing of the arteries.

Dialysis access may have become difficult over the years, leading to frequent hospital admissions. Older patients may also have been bereaved due to the death of their spouse, resulting in less motivation to carry on for the sake of others. Whatever the reasons, the person may feel that it is no longer worth the struggle to continue.

If a patient asks renal unit staff to discontinue dialysis, the subject should be gently explored, to see whether there is anything that can be done to improve the situation. In some people, the request to withdraw is a cry for help, or an expression of a state of depression that could be helped either by counselling or by medication. In some cases, patients may be asked to talk things over with a counsellor, psychologist or psychiatrist.

Stopping dialysis is a decision that should not be rushed, but properly considered. Some patients wish to stop, but find their families become distressed by the suggestion. It is important that the feelings of the others who are involved are considered and explored, but the final decision should rest with the patient.

Withdrawing from treatment after a kidney transplant

While a successful transplant offers the best possible quality of life for a patient with kidney failure, it is not without risks. The powerful drugs used to prevent rejection can lead to infections, skin cancers and, in a minority of cases, more serious cancers, especially lymphoma.

Patients need to be aware of the risks as well as the benefits of transplantation and to discuss concerns with their consultant.

One of the treatments for some serious types of cancer (including lymphoma) is to stop or reduce the doses of the immunosuppressant drugs. In this case, the kidney may be rejected, and the patient will need to go back onto dialysis. If the cancer is so advanced that no measures will prevent it, the patient is left with a bleak decision. Life might be prolonged for a short time by stopping the immunosuppressant drugs and returning to dialysis. But this involves more time spent in hospital when time is already short. The advantage of being on dialysis is that the patient can choose when they've had enough and decide to withdraw. Some patients, however, feel it is preferable to continue the immunosuppressant drugs and maintain the kidney, but allow the cancer to take a quicker course. Should you be unlucky enough to find yourself in this situation, your doctors should be able to guide you as to the best decision in your particular case.

There is another group of patients, often the elderly, who build up serious (though not fatal) complications of kidney failure, such as bone pain or 'dialysis access' problems. These complications can become too much for them. They can take the opportunity of their transplant's natural failure to allow themselves to die. This is more common when the patient is not fit enough to have another transplant.

Death from kidney failure

One of the most common questions patients and their loved ones ask is about dying from kidney failure. Many patients are concerned about dying, particularly if they have chosen not to have dialysis (conservative care) or if they are stopping treatment. It can seem difficult to talk to renal unit staff, whose lives are devoted to maintaining life, about what it is like to die from kidney failure. While every death is different (just as every life is different), in general, it can be pain-free and peaceful. The problems that occur in the final days of life vary from person to person. The symptoms that may need to be controlled include feeling sick (nausea), muscle twitching and breathlessness. Sometimes patients may become agitated, distressed and confused. Pain is not usually a serious problem.

Nausea can be caused by the waste products, usually removed by normal kidneys, building up in the blood. There are several drugs available that can be used to reduce or prevent nausea.

Breathlessness may be due to fluid overload but is not normally a problem with careful fluid management. Drugs can ensure that an individual patient is comfortable and free from distress, although most of the drugs used for nausea, breathlessness or distress (e.g. morphine and similar drugs) cause sedation, leading to some drowsiness.

Patients and families usually want to know how long a person can survive with untreated established renal failure (ERF). This is different for every patient, depending on how much their kidneys are working – and therefore the amount of urine that they pass. The kidneys may be able to get rid of some excess fluid, but unable to process waste products such as creatinine and urea, or salts such as potassium.

It is the build-up of these substances in the blood (especially the potassium) that usually leads to death.

On average, patients who are passing sufficient amounts of urine (say, over 1 litre per day) can survive for about 2–6 weeks. If little or no urine is passed, they may survive for 10–14 days. During this period, they become increasingly weak and drowsy, sleep more and more, and finally become unconscious. Then they will pass away peacefully.

When is this important?

Death is inevitable for all of us, so it is important that people talk about it. When you are discussing the pros and cons of treatment in the first place, it may be that you decide that dialysis is not what you want. It may be that when you are on dialysis, the burden of treatment is too much, and you want to stop. It could be that something changes medically that changes your priorities. You might develop another medical problem – for example, a stroke or some form of cancer – that affects your dialysis treatment. You may have a view about whether you would want to be resuscitated if your heart stopped. Thinking about these issues is very important and should be regularly reviewed by you and your team.

End of life care

An end of life care plan can help patients to decide where they would like to die; either at home, in hospital or in a hospice. Everyone involved will then make every effort to make sure that the patient's wishes are met and that their death is pain-free, dignified and in the place of their choosing.

Legal issues
Those who cannot make an informed choice

Some patients may have a condition or illness that makes it impossible for them to be in a position to choose what they wish to do. Those with advanced dementia (Alzheimer's disease, for example) or severe learning difficulties may not be able to understand the implications of the decision. They might, in addition, be unable to understand the necessity of attending for dialysis, or of being on a special diet and fluid restriction – and would find the treatment very hard to tolerate.

People who have had a stroke causing irreversible brain damage cannot express an opinion about their wishes. In such cases, it is much more difficult for the doctors to know how to act in the patient's best interests. It can be helpful, especially for the relatives, if people with kidney failure make their wishes known at a time when they are able to decide for themselves.

If you feel that there are circumstances in which you would not wish to be kept alive by dialysis, you can confirm this in writing, and ask for the document to be kept in your medical notes. A 'Living Will', an 'Advance Directive' or an 'Advance Decision' can be valuable to make sure others, including doctors, know your wishes about your health and care. Drawing one up can provide reassurance in case a time comes when you cannot make choices and decisions yourself.

If you prepare an Advance Decision according to the requirements of the Mental Capacity Act 2005, the doctors who are looking after you must legally follow your wishes. This is the case even if they do not believe it is in your best interests.

If you do not want to receive life-saving treatment (dialysis or a transplant), your Advance Decision must be put into writing. It needs to be signed and witnessed, and say clearly that you wish your directions to be followed, even if your life is at risk. An Advance Decision document will only be used if you no longer have the capacity to make the decision yourself.

Different laws apply in England and Wales to those in Northern Ireland and Scotland, so it's important to find out how these may affect a living will, depending on where you live.

Consent, capacity and best interest

It is worth covering a little bit of the legalities of the consent laws in the UK. The Mental Capacity Act (MCA) 2005 states that the only person who can consent to treatment (for adults) is the person themself. In all other cases, the clinical team, guided by others, must act in the best interests of the individual they are looking after.

In most cases, this is never a problem. Most people are perfectly able to give or withhold consent and even if the medical team disagrees with that decision, they must abide by it.

However, every time consent is needed, the 'capacity' of the individual must be considered. The process that medical teams follow is to ask whether the person has a medical problem that is preventing them consenting. If possible, the medical problem should be treated. It might be that the person is confused because they have an infection or they have low blood sugar. In that sort of situation (and provided there are no other emergencies) the team should treat and reverse that problem. If there is no medical problem, then the individual is deemed to have consent and they are in charge of any decisions.

It is important to note that someone can withdraw their consent to treatment at any time. Also, the patient's 'capacity' may change depending on the decision itself and in different circumstances.

If, however, the problem cannot be treated, or cannot be treated in a timely way, the most senior clinician should answer some further questions to work out whether the person can make a decision at the moment it is needed. The questions that need to be considered are:

1 Does the person understand the decision?
2 Can they retain the information long enough to make a decision?
3 Can they weigh up the facts? and finally
4 Can they communicate their decision to other people?

If any of those are answered by no, then the person is deemed not to have the capacity to consent under the MCA 2005. The team must then act in the best interests of the individual using their clinical judgement and the support and advice from others, such as friends and relatives. Three important statements of intent are:

1 **Advance Decisions.** Has an Advance Decision to refuse treatment been made about the decision in question (only in relation to the healthcare decision) and is it still relevant?
2 **Lasting Power of Attorney.** Is a Lasting Power of Attorney (LPA) in place for the decision in question?
3 **Court of Protection Deputy.** Has any deputy been appointed by the Court of Protection for the decision in question?

In these three cases the instruction of that legally binding decision should be followed.

Otherwise the medical team must access as much additional information as possible. For example, the person may have written a statement when they had capacity, indicated their wishes to family, friends and carers, or may have beliefs and values likely to influence their attitude to the decision, e.g. religious, cultural, lifestyle choices.

The Act places a duty on the decision maker to discuss the situation with anyone with an interest in the care of the patient who lacks capacity. This might include people the patient has nominated in the past, other professionals, such as a GP or social worker, and family and friends.

Once these processes have been completed the team can then act in the best interests of the individual.

Advanced kidney failure can affect the ability of someone to reason, yet it is reversible. So by making intentions clear through an advance directive everyone knows the plan. We would strongly encourage people to think about the difficult and complex decisions that are involved in dialysis and communicate them ahead of time. The team want to do what you want.

Where should the last days be spent?

It is very important for some people to feel they are in familiar surroundings, with family members and pets around them.

Some hospices will admit kidney patients who have decided to stop dialysis or not to start it in the first place. Hospice care and support of the dying is very sympathetic, considering the needs and feelings of both patient and family.

Most kidney units are experienced in the care of dying patients, who are usually nursed in a side ward, offering quiet and privacy. It is usual for relatives to be allowed to stay with the patient all the time. Some kidney units offer accommodation in a 'relatives' room'. One of the benefits of remaining in hospital is that, if the person has a change of heart and decides to go for dialysis, the facilities are close at hand.

Spiritual concerns

Those who do not wish to have dialysis, or would like to stop treatment, sometimes express concerns that this is the equivalent of suicide, and therefore against the teachings of most major religions. The same views might also be expressed by patients who allow their transplants to fail and then refuse dialysis. However, leaders from a number of different faiths have considered the case of the kidney patient who wishes to withdraw from treatment. None has concluded that such withdrawal is either suicidal or sinful. The basis for this is that, but for an artificial and highly technological treatment, the patient would have died naturally in the first place. As a result of human intervention, the patient has lived beyond his or her natural term. To give up dialysis or stop taking immunosuppressant drugs is simply to cease prolonging life unnaturally in someone whose body is not capable of sustaining itself.

Any patient, or relative of a patient, who has any concerns or needs spiritual support should talk to his or her priest or religious leader. Many hospitals have a chaplaincy service, with leaders from all the major faiths available to give support and advice.

KEY FACTS

1 Dialysis is not compulsory. A trial of treatment may be a sensible option, while you are making up your mind.

2 Withdrawal from dialysis is not uncommon, especially in older patients.

3 The reason for withdrawal from treatment is usually a medical event unrelated to the kidneys, such as a stroke or cancer.

4 The decision should not be rushed, allowing time for others to come to terms with the situation.

5 Conservative care, or conservative management, is the term used when patients have decided that they don't want dialysis or a transplant.

6 People who have conservative care will be given medicines to control their symptoms.

7 If treatment for kidney failure is not taken when it's needed, the patient will die. This usually happens within a few days or weeks.

8 Death from renal failure need not be distressing, if well managed. It should take place where the patient feels most comfortable.

9 The wish to stop dialysis may be due to depression, or a cry for help, needing action to improve some intolerable situation.

10 Kidney patients have greater control in ensuring a dignified death than most other people.

11 Preparing an Advance Decision may be useful if you know that you would not want to continue treatment if you lost your mental capacity to make decisions.

12 Transplant patients can decide to stop their immunosuppressant drugs, to make them reject and lose the kidney, and then not have dialysis. In this way, they can allow themselves to die of kidney failure.

13 Refusing dialysis, or deliberately allowing a transplant to fail, is not suicide.

14 If religion is important to a patient, it is a good idea for them to discuss these issues with a priest or other religious leader – either from their own community or from the hospital.

SECTION 3:

Reference material – complications, tests and other information

11 FLUID BALANCE

This chapter describes how the amount of fluid in the body is controlled by healthy kidneys. It looks at the problem of too much or too little fluid in the body when kidneys fail. It also gives information on how to manage the levels of water in the body when kidneys no longer work properly.

Introduction

One of the two main functions of the kidneys is to remove excess fluid from the body. Fluid comes into the body from drinks, and also from food, especially high-liquid food such as juicy fruit, soup, jelly and ice-cream. By removing excess fluid from the body, the kidneys are able to control the body's fluid content. This is called fluid balance. To understand fluid balance, it helps to know a bit about how the body is made up.

Flesh and fluid

The body is made up of two main parts: flesh and fluid. The flesh is all the solid parts of the body, such as bone, muscle and fat. Most of the fluid part is simply water and salts (for example Sodium Chloride) such as in the blood, urine and saliva. Men have approximately 60% of fluid to 40% of flesh in their bodies, whereas women, whose bodies contain a higher proportion of fat, have approximately 55% of fluid to 45% of flesh (see Figure 11.1).

Changes in your fluid 'balance' are easier to see. The easiest way to see a change in the amount of fluid in the body is to measure body weight. The known weight of 1 litre of water is 1 kilogram. So, if you weigh yourself, then drink 1 litre of water, then weigh yourself again, your weight should show an increase of about 1 kilogram. The weight increase is instant.

In contrast, flesh weight changes more gradually. It is more difficult to see a change in flesh weight because when a person's flesh weight goes up (usually because they have eaten food that has a lot of calories), it does not happen immediately. For example, if you ate two big cream doughnuts and weighed yourself immediately afterwards, you may not see very much difference. Flesh weight tends to change over a much longer period of time.

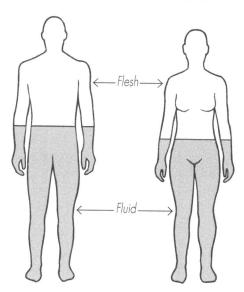

Figure 11.1: Fluid and flesh proportions in the human body

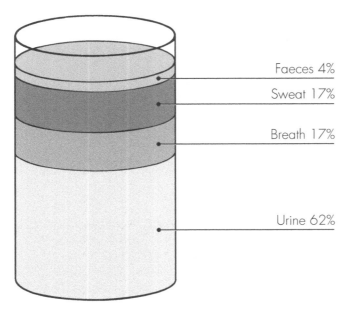

Faeces 4%

Sweat 17%

Breath 17%

Urine 62%

Figure 11.2: Fluid loss from the human body

Control of fluid balance

Normal healthy kidneys can easily control the amount of fluid in the body. If you do not have kidney failure, you do not have to think about your fluid balance because your kidneys control the amount of urine you pass.

If a person drinks ten pints of water (or beer), they will usually pass a little less than ten pints of urine. Similarly, if they drink three cups of tea per day, they can expect to pass the equivalent of just under three teacups of urine.

The small difference is because fluid is also lost from the body in other ways – as you breathe, when you sweat and in your faeces (see Figure 11.2). If someone becomes very hot, they will sweat more. To control fluid balance, they will then need to offset the fluid lost in sweat by passing less urine.

In kidney failure, it is different. Many people with failing kidneys do not pass any urine at all. Others pass exactly the same amount of urine every day, no matter how much they drink. This means these patients are unable to control how much water is in the body. If someone with kidney failure drinks too much, they may keep that fluid in their body. This is called fluid overload. Conversely, if someone with kidney failure drinks too little, or loses too much fluid from the body (say, through sweating), they will become dehydrated. Finding the balance is not always easy.

What is the 'target weight'?

The term 'target weight' means the weight that the doctor considers to be the 'best' weight for an individual patient. At this weight, there will be neither too much nor too little fluid in the body. This target weight may change over time. A kidney patient's target weight may have to go up or down as flesh weight is gained or lost. Flesh weight increases if a person eats too much, or may decrease due to dieting or illness. Getting the target weight may also require a little trial and error. The team may use the blood pressure to help with this process, or ask about symptoms of cramp when on haemodialysis.

Weight also changes according to how much fluid is in the body. If a person has too much fluid in their body (i.e. is fluid overloaded, see below), they will weigh more. This is very important when someone is receiving dialysis. If you are above your 'target weight' that is telling you that you have too much salt and water in your body and that needs to be removed, normally through dialysis. This is particularly relevant if you need haemodialysis. Each time you need a session you will need weighing and the difference between your target weight and your measured weight will be the amount of fluid that needs removing. That difference (for haemodialysis) is called the 'intradialytic weight gain' – since it is the fluid built up between sessions. This needs to be kept as low as possible to protect your heart (see Chapter 5).

The target weight, therefore, is the ideal weight when the person is neither 'wet' (fluid overloaded) nor 'dry' (dehydrated). Other names for target weight are 'dry' weight or 'ideal' weight.

Sodium (salt) and fluid balance

Sodium (salt) is a mineral that plays a part in helping to control the body's fluid balance. Too much salt makes us thirsty and can contribute to high blood pressure. People who have kidney failure, especially those who are on dialysis, should avoid eating salty foods and adding salt to their food either at the table or in cooking.

Salt is found in very many foods. It is often easy to see which food contains salt, for example crisps and salted nuts. However salt is hidden in many processed foods too, so it's important to read the labels on food packaging and check the salt (or sodium) content.

Remember, eating salty foods makes people want to drink more fluid. If people with kidney failure drink too much, they may develop fluid overload.

Fluid overload

What is fluid overload and why does it matter?

Fluid overload is a condition in which there is too much fluid in the body. It is caused by drinking too much fluid, or by the body not removing enough. Fluid overload also causes (or worsens) high blood pressure (see Chapter 12).

When the fluid content of the body reaches a very high level, excess fluid collects in and under the skin. There are no early signs of fluid overload but it usually first shows as swelling around the ankles. This is called ankle oedema. The reason the ankles are affected first is simple – gravity tends to make fluid fall to the bottom of the body.

If fluid overload is not treated, the swelling due to excess fluid slowly creeps up the body into the thighs, and then into the lower abdomen and lower back. If it is not treated, fluid will continue to spread up the body, and eventually settle in the lungs. Fluid in the lungs, which causes shortness of breath, is called pulmonary oedema. This is a very serious condition which can be life-threatening.

Occasionally, people with kidney failure suddenly develop pulmonary oedema, without going through the 'warning stages' of ankle and leg swelling. This can happen if they drink a lot of fluid very quickly. When pulmonary oedema comes on this quickly, it needs urgent treatment. And urgent means exactly that – treatment straight away!

Fluid overload happens mainly to kidney patients on dialysis. However, it can be a problem for pre-dialysis patients too, and also for people who have had a kidney transplant.

How is fluid overload treated?

Remember, 'what goes in has to come out'. Therefore the first treatment of fluid overload for all people with kidney failure is simply to drink less. However, this is not usually enough. It is also important that they cut down on salt in their diet, since salt increases thirst. Additional treatments depend on whether or not the kidneys are still making urine, often referred to as having residual renal function (RRF).

1 **Patients with residual renal function.** If patients are pre-dialysis, if they have a failing transplant, or if they are on dialysis and still pass some urine, they will usually be given tablets called diuretics ('water tablets') to treat fluid overload. The tablets work by increasing the amount of urine that is passed every day. A combination of passing more urine and drinking less usually does the trick. Two commonly used diuretic drugs are furosemide and bumetanide. Stronger diuretics, such as metolazone, may be given as well.

   If taking diuretics and drinking less does not get rid of all the fluid, it may be necessary for patients not already doing so, to have dialysis.

2 **Patients with no residual renal function.** Everyone without residual renal function requires dialysis. Dialysis patients who get fluid overload should also drink less. However, diuretics don't normally work and so a different treatment for fluid overload is needed. These patients need a combination of drinking less (usually a daily limit of 0.5 to 1 litre for haemodialysis patients and 0.5 to 1.5 litres for PD patients), and removing more fluid by dialysis.

It sounds easy to 'drink less', however many people find it very difficult to manage. Our lives often focus on activities that involve drinking, such as meeting friends for a coffee, going to the pub or going out for a meal. Drinking is a sociable thing to do and it can be hard to avoid. However, there are some tricks and tips that many people find useful, such as using a small cup to drink out of; sucking ice cubes (but don't forget this is water too) and cleaning your teeth or using mouthwash to stop the feeling of thirst. Also, chewing sugar free gum or sucking sugar free sweets can also help.

You can also help yourself by not eating salt or salty food, spreading your drinks throughout the day and keeping a record of how much you have had to drink. And remember, food also contains fluid – soup is mainly liquid, and water melon is very aptly named.

Protein and fluid balance

Protein comes from the food we eat (such as meat, fish and eggs) and is digested in the gut before entering the bloodstream. Protein plays a big part in balancing fluid in the body. It helps the fluid move out from the body's tissues and under the skin (such as swollen ankles, legs and hands) and into the bloodstream so that it can be removed by the kidneys (in urine) or by dialysis.

If there isn't enough protein in the body, any excess fluid will remain in the tissues, and the treatments for fluid overload will not work.

Dehydration

Dehydration is the opposite of fluid overload. It occurs when there is too little fluid in the body. Dehydration may occur if someone does not drink enough, or if they lose fluid as a result of sweating, diarrhoea or vomiting. Sometimes, people can get dehydrated when they have had a kidney transplant if they do not drink enough.

It can be difficult for people to judge when they are dehydrated. However, dehydration is almost always accompanied by low blood pressure. This is easier to identify than high blood pressure. Low blood pressure makes people feel weak and dizzy when they stand up.

How is dehydration treated?

Any patient with kidney failure who is suffering from dehydration needs to drink more. If a patient (pre-dialysis or with a failing transplant) takes diuretics, these should be reduced or stopped. If the dehydration is severe, admission to hospital for intravenous fluids (via a drip) may be necessary. For dialysis patients, a reduction in the amount of water removed by dialysis may be needed. If haemodialysis patients are severely dehydrated, they can be given fluid during a dialysis session by intravenous infusion (directly into the blood).

Taking control of your own fluid balance

Keeping the right balance of fluid in your body is crucial for long-term health when you have kidney failure. This is particularly important if you have haemodialysis as the dialysis is not done every day and body fluid will build up between treatments.

Keeping the right balance means making sure that the amount you drink is no more than the amount of fluid that is removed by dialysis. You are in control of how much you drink, and can learn to judge how much is safe for you.

KEY FACTS

1   Fluid balance is the balance between fluid coming into the body, from drinks and food, and fluid leaving the body, mainly in the urine or by dialysis.

2   Fluid = Salts such as sodium and water.

3   Too much fluid in the body is called fluid overload. This may cause swelling of the ankles.

4   If you eat salty foods, such as bacon, crisps and many pre-packed foods, you will become very thirsty and will probably drink more. So control of salt intake is vital for control of fluid balance.

5   The treatment of fluid overload is to drink less, and to remove more fluid from the body. This is done by taking diuretics (water tablets), or by increasing the amount of water removed by dialysis.

6   If fluid overload is not treated, shortness of breath due to fluid in the lungs may develop. This condition – known as pulmonary oedema – needs urgent treatment in hospital.

7   Judging the amount of fluid in the body is difficult. But, with practice, patients can learn to 'feel' when they are on their target weight – i.e. when they are neither 'wet' (fluid overloaded) nor 'dry' (dehydrated).

8   When there is too little water in the body (dehydration), dizziness may occur.

9   The treatment of dehydration is to drink more, and to remove less fluid from the body. This is done either by stopping diuretics, or by reducing the amount of fluid removed by dialysis.

10 Fluid balance is one area where you can really take control and do a lot to help yourself. Make sure that the amount you drink is no more than the amount of fluid that can be removed by dialysis. Learn to judge how much is safe for you. Help yourself by avoiding salty food that makes you thirsty. Use a small cup to drink out of and spreading your drinks throughout the day.

12 BLOOD PRESSURE

This chapter looks at the link between blood pressure and kidney failure. It also explains the importance of blood pressure control and how this is achieved.

Introduction

The control of blood pressure (BP) is one of the important 'extra' functions performed by the kidneys. The term 'blood pressure' means the pressure of the blood on the artery walls which are the tubes that carry blood around the body. This pressure goes up and down as the heart continuously squeezes and relaxes to pump blood around the body.

Circulation of the blood

The main function of the blood (and the blood vessels through which it flows) is to carry things around the body. Blood carries 'good things' to parts of the body where they are needed, and also removes 'bad things' so they can be got rid of, mainly by the kidneys via the urine.

Adults have about 5 litres (10 pints) of blood travelling around their body all the time. The heart acts as a pump to drive the blood through the blood vessels. There are two main types of blood vessel: arteries and veins. The arteries take blood that is rich in oxygen from the heart to all parts of the body. This oxygen, combined with the food that is eaten, provides the different parts of the body with the energy they need to do their work. The veins then take the blood (now with most of its oxygen used up) back to the heart. From there, the blood goes to the lungs to get more oxygen. It then goes back to the heart, and so the process goes on, as illustrated in Figure 12.1.

Measuring blood pressure

The blood pressure is measured using a piece of equipment known as a sphygmomanometer (or sphyg, pronounced 'sfig'). There are various different types of sphygmomanometer, but all of them measure blood pressure in units of millimetres of mercury (mmHg).

Two readings are taken. The first reading shows the pressure of the blood when the heart squeezes, and is called the systolic blood pressure. The second reading is the pressure of the blood when the heart is relaxed between squeezes. This is called the diastolic blood pressure.

The systolic pressure is always higher than the diastolic pressure, and is always recorded first. For example; a blood pressure of 130/80 mmHg (known as '130 over 80') means that the systolic pressure is 130 and the diastolic pressure is 80. A reading of 130 mmHg means that the pressure of the blood is enough to push mercury (the chemical symbol is Hg) up a column to a height of 130 millimetres.

What is 'normal' blood pressure?

There is no such thing as normal blood pressure. For most people with kidney failure, however, doctors accept a level of 130/80 or below as satisfactory. This is for patients who are not yet on dialysis, those on PD or with a transplant. The best blood pressure for a patient on haemodialysis is less clear. This is because the amount of salt and water in

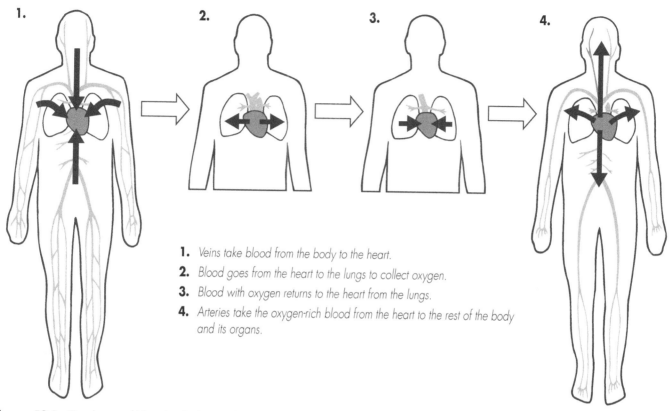

1. Veins take blood from the body to the heart.
2. Blood goes from the heart to the lungs to collect oxygen.
3. Blood with oxygen returns to the heart from the lungs.
4. Arteries take the oxygen-rich blood from the heart to the rest of the body and its organs.

Figure 12.1: Circulation of blood in the human body

the body changes massively before, during and after each HD session. However, the aim is for all patients to have a blood pressure similar to the ideal level.

The blood pressure varies continuously throughout the heart's pumping cycle. This means that during each cycle, the systolic blood pressure is, say, 140 or 180 for only a fraction of a second. Blood pressure also varies according to the time of day – tending to be higher in the morning and again in the early evening. And there is a difference between one arm and the other. Slight variations may also result from using different sphygmomanometers, or from how different people use the same piece of equipment.

If there is doubt about whether or not a patient has

high blood pressure, a 24-hour blood pressure test can be organised. This involves a patient carrying a cuff on their arm for 24 hours. Every hour, the cuff automatically inflates and deflates, giving the doctor a better idea of the average blood pressure over the 24-hour period.

High blood pressure and kidney failure

High blood pressure is very common in people with kidney failure. The connection between these two conditions is two-way. High blood pressure can cause kidney failure, and kidney failure causes high blood pressure. It is often difficult to know for certain whether a patient's high blood pressure has caused their kidney failure, or whether kidney failure has caused their high blood pressure.

High blood pressure can occur in kidney patients who are pre-dialysis, who are on dialysis, or who have had a transplant. Many patients with kidney failure are taking one, two or even three types of blood pressure tablet.

Many patients with kidney failure have to take an injection treatment called erythropoietin stimulating agent (ESA) for anaemia (see Chapter 7). If you have high blood pressure, this treatment can make it worse. It is better, however, to stay on the ESA drug if you need it, and to take more blood pressure tablets, than to stop ESA treatment.

Low blood pressure and kidney failure

Some people with kidney failure have a different blood pressure problem. Their blood pressure is lower than it should be. Low blood pressure is usually less serious than high blood pressure, but it also needs to be treated. Very low blood pressure can be serious, though. It can be a sign that the heart is not pumping well (heart failure), or that there is fluid in the sac around the heart (pericardial effusion). Both can be treated, either by drinking more or by changing the dose or type of medicines used to treat high blood pressure.

Anxiety and blood pressure or 'white coat hypertension'

White coat hypertension is a term used to describe the elevation in BP seen when people have their blood pressure measured by a doctor or other healthcare practitioner. It is not clear why it happens, and it is not just 'anxiety', but it is common – about one in three people have it. The problem is that it can affect the way your blood pressure is treated.

Anxiety is not a major factor in high blood pressure. Although anxiety can put the blood pressure up a little,

it is a mistake to blame repeated high blood pressure readings on, for example, 'the stress of the journey' or a 'fear of seeing the doctor', or even 'difficulty parking'. So in these cases blood pressure needs to be measured with a 24-hour monitor or by doing it yourself.

How do you know that your blood pressure is high or low?

There are no reliable symptoms of high or low blood pressure so the only reliable way of finding out what your blood pressure is, is to have it measured. Some people with very high blood pressure suffer from headaches but that is uncommon. But the fact that you do not have headaches does not mean that you do not have high blood pressure.

One of the symptoms of low blood pressure is dizziness, especially when you stand up. However, people can experience dizzy spells for other reasons. If you do feel dizzy, it is important to check your blood pressure to make sure it isn't low.

You cannot rely on your body to tell you if your blood pressure is low or high. You have to have your blood pressure checked.

What determines blood pressure levels?

A person's blood pressure is affected by the following important factors:

1 **The amount of salt and water in the body.** If there is too much salt and water in the body (fluid overload), the blood pressure will go up. If there is too little salt and water in the body (dehydration), the blood pressure will go down. (Both fluid overload and dehydration, and their treatments, are described in Chapter 11.) People who have kidney failure and cannot easily balance the amount of water in their body are therefore at risk of high or low blood pressure.

2 **The 'suppleness' or 'flexibility' of the arteries.** The arteries are constantly changing in width as blood

flows through them. So, it's important for them to be supple and flexible to allow them to react to how your body is working. The narrower and harder the arteries become, the higher the blood pressure will go. Narrow and hard arteries can be caused by a build-up of cholesterol or calcium inside the blood vessels. The most common causes of this build-up are smoking or eating a high fat diet and being overweight. Smoking also causes narrowing of the arteries.

3 **How well the heart works.** The strength of contraction of the heart, and the rate it beats, also affect blood pressure. Generally speaking, the harder or faster the heart beats, the higher the blood pressure will be.

Why treat high blood pressure?

There are several important reasons to treat high blood pressure. However, there is little point in treating someone for high blood pressure unless the related problems of high cholesterol levels in the blood, being overweight and smoking are also addressed. All these factors worsen the effects of high blood pressure.

High blood pressure increases the likelihood of a stroke or a heart attack by damaging the blood vessels.

There are also 'kidney reasons' to treat high blood pressure. If blood pressure is high for a period of time, a patient with kidney failure may have to start dialysis sooner than would otherwise be necessary. This is because uncontrolled high blood pressure can speed up damage to the kidneys. In fact, controlling blood pressure is the only thing proven to delay the need for dialysis in all kidney patients, whatever the cause of their kidney failure.

Good blood pressure control may not stop the need dialysis, but it can mean that dialysis does not need to be started so soon. It may also help to keep a kidney transplant working well for longer.

How is high blood pressure treated?

High blood pressure can be treated by making changes to your lifestyle that improve the circulation of blood around your body and by taking medicines which:

a Increase the width of the arteries ('vasodilator' drugs);

b Reduce the strength of contraction of the heart, and the rate at which it beats (beta-blocker drugs);

c Act directly on the kidney to lower the blood pressure (ACE inhibitor drugs and ARB drugs);

d Remove excess water from the body (Loop diuretics and thiazides drugs);

e Act on the body's blood pressure control signals (centrally acting antihypertensive drugs).

More detailed information about these treatments can be found in Chapter 7 (Drug treatments for BP, anaemia and bones).

Lifestyle (diet, exercise and smoking)

By living a healthy lifestyle, your blood pressure can be reduced quite a lot and will certainly mean that you don't need to take as many medicines. Being overweight, being unfit and smoking all have a big impact on your blood pressure and your heart health. Making the changes outlined below can reduce your blood pressure quite quickly.

There are three things that you can do to make a difference to your blood pressure. These are eating a healthy diet, taking regular exercise and by not smoking.

Eating a healthy diet

As described in Chapter 8, a healthy diet is very important for people with kidney failure. One of the main reasons for this is that it can really help to keep your blood pressure under control. There are two parts of the diet that will have an effect on your blood pressure:

• **Salt.** It is very important for people with kidney failure to cut down on salt. Salt will make you thirsty, which will make you drink more. Taking in too much fluid will cause fluid overload, which in turn will raise your blood pressure. The excess fluid enters your bloodstream, increasing the pressure inside the blood vessels. So cutting down on salt will help to keep your fluid balance in control and in turn, keep your blood pressure down. Salt can be reduced in your diet by avoiding salty food such as crisps, ready-meals and processed food, and by not adding salt when cooking or to your meal at the table. Salt substitutes (such as Lo-Salt) should not be used as these usually are high in potassium which can be dangerous for kidney patients.

- **Weight.** Keeping your weight healthy will also keep your blood pressure down. Being overweight affects your blood pressure. People who are overweight have a build-up of a waxy substance called plaque on the inside of their blood vessels. This puts extra pressure on them, making it difficult for blood to flow around the body and so, increasing the blood pressure. So, reducing the amount of fatty and sugary food in your diet will help to keep your weight under control and reduce the risks of high blood pressure.

Taking regular exercise

As described in Chapter 2, exercise is very important for everyone, but especially people who have a long term illness such as kidney disease. Becoming more active will not only help reduce your blood pressure, but it will also help improve your mood and increase your energy levels. For advice on exercise take a look at Chapter 8.

Stopping Smoking

Smoking cigarettes and pipe tobacco can affect your blood pressure in two ways. Firstly, each time you smoke a cigarette, the blood pressure goes up temporarily. Secondly, smoking will cause fatty substances to build up inside your arteries. This narrows the blood vessel and causes pressure to rise. There is a lot of help available to help you to stop smoking. Talk to your doctor at the hospital or your GP or practice nurse. The pharmacist at your local chemist may also be able to help. There are also support groups that may be useful to join. If you find it very hard to stop, you may be offered counselling, nicotine replacement therapy (NRT) with nicotine patches or gum, or medication.

Taking control of your own blood pressure

High blood pressure is not something you just need to 'suffer' with. The three golden rules for keeping your blood pressure down are:

- take your blood pressure tablets;
- don't get fluid-overloaded;
- don't eat too much salt;
- take exercise and keep your weight at a sensible level.

If you are asked to take your own blood pressure it is important that you always do it in the same way and keep a record to show the doctors and nurses when you visit the clinic. Most people find it easiest to use the electronic blood pressure machines that can easily be bought from chemist shops. They are not too expensive and can really help you to manage your blood pressure. Ensure you get a machine approved by the British Hypertension Society (http://bhsoc.org/bp-monitors/bp-monitors). You should always:

- Make sure you are calm when you take your blood pressure. Sit down and rest for about 5 minutes before you take the reading.
- Put the blood pressure cuff on the same arm each time you take you blood pressure.
- Take the recording at a similar time of day each time; for example always do it in the morning, or at night-time.
- Try to have the blood pressure machine at the same height as your heart when you take the reading. This is easily done if you sit down when you are taking your blood pressure and put the machine on a table.
- Keep still and silent while your blood pressure is being taken.
- Take the reading three times and use the lowest reading.

- Make a note of the reading in a notebook, or on your smartphone. Write down the reading exactly as it is shown on the machine. Do not round the numbers up or down.

KEY FACTS

1 High blood pressure is very common in people with kidney failure.

2 An acceptable blood pressure will be 130/80 or below, for most people.

3 Kidney failure causes high blood pressure, and high blood pressure causes kidney failure.

4 The injection treatment for anaemia, called erythropoietin stimulating agents (ESAs), can increase your blood pressure.

5 High blood pressure also increases the likelihood of a stroke or heart attack.

6 You cannot reliably 'feel' your own blood pressure, especially when it is high. You have to have it checked.

7 High blood pressure can be controlled by removing fluid from your body and by taking blood pressure tablets.

8 Too much salt in the diet may make the blood pressure higher.

9 You have the opportunity to take a large part of responsibility for controlling your own blood pressure. Have it checked regularly, don't drink too much fluid, avoid salt wherever possible, and make sure you take the tablets your doctor prescribes for you.

10 If you are asked to take your own blood pressure, do it in the same way each time and keep a record.

13 REFERENCE GUIDE

These pages give you a guide to the most common blood tests you will have taken. Know about these 10 tests and you will cover 80% of the tests you will have as a routine.

Introduction

The information in this chapter serves as a handy reference guide, but if you have detailed questions about your results discuss the issues with your GP or renal team. You may notice that there are few stated 'normal ranges'. This is because different labs often have different normal values for these tests, depending on the type of test they use.

'Normal' may also vary according to your sex or age. So ask your doctor for the normal range or check on Patient View. For some of the tests, we have given the recommended levels based on the guidance of NICE and the Renal Association.

A full guide can be found at http://labtestsonline.org.uk/map/aindex

The blood tests covered here are the basic ones you will see on Patient View and will give you a good idea of your clinical state. There are many others – ask your team.

BLOOD: YOUR TOP 10!	
1	Creatinine
2	eGFR
3	Haemoglobin
4	Ferritin
5	Potassium
6	Albumin
7	Phosphate
8	Calcium
9	PTH
10	C-reactive protein

Creatinine
What is it?

Creatinine is a waste product produced in your muscles from the breakdown of a compound called creatine which is made as your muscles work. Creatinine is excreted by the kidneys, so blood concentrations measure how well your kidneys are working. The lower your serum creatinine the better your kidney function, but ask your doctor what the normal values are for your laboratory.

The quantity produced depends on the sex, size or age of the person and their muscle mass, as well as how much protein they consume. So creatinine concentrations will be higher in people with more muscle bulk than in smaller people.

NICE guidelines advise people not to eat any meat in the 12 hours before having a blood test for creatinine. This will help give a more accurate test result.

Why is it important?

It is used to judge how well your kidneys are working and is used to calculate a test result called estimated Glomerular Filtration Rate (eGFR). In people on dialysis it can be used to determine how effective the dialysis is since creatinine is removed by dialysis treatment. It is not directly toxic.

What can be done about it?

Nothing needs to be done about it but it is used to monitor changes in kidney function.

Estimated Glomerular Filtration Rate (eGFR)
What is it?

The glomerular filtration rate is the amount of blood (measured in ml) that the kidneys filter in a minute. Since the normal value is about 100, you may hear people talk about it as % kidney function, although that is not strictly accurate. Measuring GFR is very complex so the creatinine test is used to calculate an estimate – this is called estimated GFR (eGFR).

This result can then be used to monitor the progress of kidney disease and to classify the stage of kidney disease (see Chapter 1, Figure 1.4).

Why is it important?

eGFR is a better way to monitor kidney function than serum creatinine, and allows your doctor to judge the severity of the kidney problem as well the rate at which it is changing. Unlike creatinine, the lower the number, the poorer the kidney function. It is not a useful measure for people on dialysis treatment.

What can be done about it?

Nothing needs to be done about eGFR, but it is used to monitor changes in kidney function. It is important to understand that there is a degree of variation in the accuracy of the test so it is better to look at several results as a trend rather than as single results. It can be used as a guide to know when to start dialysis – in the UK people start dialysis with an average eGFR of 8.5 mls/min/1.73m2 – but it should not be the only measure used. There are lots of things that are taken into consideration when deciding whether a patient needs to start treatment – including other blood tests and symptoms.

Haemoglobin

- Normal range varies by age and sex but is in the range 120–180 g/L.
- Recommended concentration for dialysis patients on EPO 100–120 g/L

What is it?

This test measures the amount of haemoglobin (a protein found in red blood cells) in your blood. Haemoglobin carries oxygen to cells from the lungs. If your haemoglobin levels are low, you have anaemia. Anaemia causes fatigue and weakness because your blood is not able to carry enough oxygen around the body.

Why is it important?

Anaemia is common in people with kidney disease and becomes more common as kidney function falls. Chapter 7 details more information about this.

What can be done about it?

Chapter 7 covers details of the different treatments for renal anaemia but includes the use of iron supplements, EPO and other ESAs and blood transfusions when absolutely needed.

Ferritin

- Ferritin is measured in nanograms (ng) per millitre. The recommended concentration for CKD and dialysis patients is 100–800 ng/ml (ideal 200–500 ng/ml).

What is it?

Iron is needed by the body to make haemoglobin that carries oxygen around the body. The body maintains stores of iron within cells. Within them, iron is stored within proteins including one called ferritin (although there are others). Ferritin is the main storage complex and is present mostly in the liver, but also in the bone marrow, spleen and muscles. Small amounts of ferritin also circulate in the blood. The ferritin concentration within the bloodstream reflects the amount of iron stored in your body.

Why is it important?

It is used to judge how much iron there is in your body. Low levels indicate a potential iron shortage. High levels can indicate too much iron but levels can also rise when there is infection or inflammation within the body.

What can be done about it?

Chapter 7 covers details of potential treatment for renal anaemia but includes the use of iron supplements, EPO and other ESAs and blood transfusions when absolutely needed.

Potassium

What is it?

Potassium is salt or electrolyte that is present throughout your body. Most potassium is stored inside your cells with a carefully regulated concentration within your blood.

Potassium has important actions that allow all muscles (including your heart) to work and for nerve cells to transmit signals.

A low concentration of potassium in the blood is called hypokalaemia and a high level is called hyperkalaemia.

What should it be?

- Normal range 3.5 – 5.2 mmol/L
- Haemodialysis 4.0 to 6.0 mmol/L
- Pre-dialysis and peritoneal dialysis – maintain in normal range

Why is it important?

Both very high and low levels can be dangerous. In extreme cases it can cause the heart to stop working without warning.

What can be done about it?

The kidneys normally regulate potassium in the blood but when they are not working well (or at all) dialysis treatment will remove it. However, dialysis is not as effective as healthy kidneys so people with kidney failure will be advised to restrict the amount of potassium in their diet. High potassium foods include fruit, chocolate and potatoes.

If the potassium concentration is low you may be asked to eat more high-potassium foods. Alternatively, potassium tablets may be prescribed.

Some tablets, including ACE inhibitors and ARBs (see Chapter 7), can cause potassium concentrations to rise. If this happens, they may need to be reduced or stopped.

Albumin

What is it?

Albumin is the most abundant protein in the blood. It carries vitamins and hormones around the body and many drugs bind to it. Some of the 'salts' of the blood, like calcium, also bind to it. It is a building block for our tissues.

Why is it important?

If kidneys leak excess protein, levels can also fall. This is seen in diseases of the kidneys that cause something called nephrotic syndrome. Low levels may be seen in advanced malnutrition but it is not a good measure of early malnutrition.

When albumin concentrations are low, fluid (salt and water) can leak out of the blood into the tissues. This can result in swollen legs. The problem here is that the fluid is in the wrong place. There is less fluid in the blood, so blood pressure can be low, yet the legs are swollen or fluid may rest in the lungs causing breathing problems.

What can be done about it?

The underlying problem needs to be treated depending on what has caused the low albumin levels. In particular, for dialysis patients, a dietitian has an important role to make sure people have enough food.

Calcium

- Recommended levels for dialysis patients – between 2.2 and 2.5 mmol/L (measured pre-dialysis in HD patients)

What is it?

Calcium is one of the most important minerals or salts in the body. Most of it is found in the bones but about 1% is circulating in the blood. Half of that is bound to proteins such as albumin. The free calcium is the active mineral in the blood. Normally labs measure the total amount of calcium in the blood (called total calcium) and may correct it for the albumin level in the blood; this measures both the active and inactive forms of calcium.

Why is it important?

A high calcium level is called hypercalcaemia. This means you have too much calcium in your blood and will need treatment for the condition that is causing this. In patients on dialysis this is either due to the medication (vitamin D or calcium-containing phosphate binders) or a very overactive parathyroid gland (tertiary hyperparathyroidism). This is covered in Chapter 7.

There are other important causes unrelated to the kidney disease. These can include cancer or an overactive thyroid gland but there are a lot of other causes your team may need to think about.

Low calcium levels, called hypocalcaemia, mean that you do not have enough calcium in your blood. This can be caused by medication such as cinacalcet or by a lack of active vitamin D in people with kidney disease.

High and low levels can cause problems with the heart and other muscles so it can be very serious. It can result in tummy pain, constipation and nausea and vomiting.

What can be done about it?

Chapter 7 summarises the treatment of renal bone disease including options for calcium.

Phosphate

- Recommended concentrations for dialysis patients: 1.1–1.7 mmol/L.

What is it?

Phosphates are essential for energy production which allows muscles and nerves to function. It is also used for bone growth. Only about 1% of total body phosphate is found within the blood. About 70% to 80% of the phosphates are combined with calcium to help form bones and teeth, about 10% are found in muscle, and about 1% is in nerve tissue. The rest is found within cells throughout the body, where it is mainly used to store energy.

Most phosphate in the body comes from dietary sources. A variety of foods (dairy products, meat, chicken and fish) contain significant amounts of phosphate. The body regulates phosphate levels in the blood by regulating how much it absorbs from the intestines and how much it excretes or conserves in the kidneys.

Why is it important?

High levels are common in dialysis patients, especially when they are not on treatment or if they have not had dietary advice. Chapter 7 contains further information on why high phosphate levels are important but it causes bone problems as well as having an effect on the blood vessels and heart in people with kidney disease.

Low levels are also harmful. They reflects a lack of available energy so can affect muscle and heart performance. Low levels can be seen when people are not eating well and in some people on more intensive dialysis treatments such as nocturnal haemodialysis.

What can be done about it?

Chapter 7 summarises treatment. For high levels, phosphate binders are commonly used along with a low phosphate diet.

Parathormone or parathyroid hormone (PTH)

- Recommended levels for dialysis patients – between 2 and 9 times the upper limit of the 'normal' range. The 'normal range' is different in different hospital labs.

What is it?

Parathyroid hormone (PTH) helps the body maintain stable amounts of calcium in the bloodstream and looks after the bones (see Chapter 7). It is part of a 'feedback loop' that includes calcium, phosphate, vitamin D and PTH itself.

PTH is produced by four parathyroid glands that are located in the neck beside the thyroid gland. Normally, these glands secrete PTH into the bloodstream in response to low blood calcium concentration. Parathyroid hormone then works in a number of ways to help raise blood calcium back to normal. It takes calcium from the body's bone, stimulates the activation of vitamin D in the kidney (which in turn increases the absorption of calcium from the intestines), reduces the excretion of calcium in the urine and increases the excretion of phosphate in the urine.

Why is it important?

High levels are common in people with end stage kidney failure. As covered in Chapter 7 this is called 'secondary hyperparathyroidism' because the glands are compensating for other problems brought about by the kidney disease. If it is left untreated it can become uncontrolled and PTH levels will rise high enough to cause the calcium level to rise – this is called 'tertiary hyperparathyroidism'.

There is another cause of high levels of PTH. This is where either a gland itself or a benign growth within one of more of the parathyroid glands secretes extra PTH and doesn't respond to calcium levels in the blood. Calcium levels then rise. This is called 'primary hyperparathyroidsim'.

High levels of PTH can weaken the bones and elevate levels of phosphate in the blood. PTH may also cause scarring and damage to the heart and reduce the responsiveness of the bone marrow to EPO.

What can be done about it?

Chapter 7 summarises the treatment of renal bone disease. PTH levels may be reduced indirectly by lowering phosphate levels, increasing calcium or providing activated vitamin D or directly by using a drug called cinacalcet. Sometimes one or more glands will need to be removed surgically.

C-reactive protein (CRP)
What is it?
C-reactive protein (CRP) is a protein made by the liver that is released into the blood within a few hours after tissue injury, the start of an infection or other inflammatory illnesses. Increased concentrations in the blood can be found with infection or sepsis, after a heart attack, and after an operation. Levels may be slightly higher than usual all the time in people on dialysis but the concentration of CRP in the blood can jump a thousand-fold in response to an infection.

The CRP blood test provides information to the doctor about whether inflammation is present and needs to be used with other evidence to reach a diagnosis.

Why is it important?
Infection is very common in people on dialysis so it can be a useful as a test to confirm a problem or pick up problems earlier.

What can be done about it?
The underlying problem needs to be treated. It is unclear why some people on dialysis have long term rises in their CRP.

14 POLICY, ORGANISING CARE AND GETTING INVOLVED

In this chapter we discuss how the care for people with kidney disease is organised and monitored. We also look at the policies and guidelines that the NHS, professional groups and the government have introduced to try to improve the lives of people with kidney failure. The chapter also explains how you can get involved and influence the care for patients in the UK.

Introduction

The care for people diagnosed with kidney failure has improved enormously over the years. Even as recently as the 1980s there were not enough services for people with kidney failure to be treated effectively. This included the number of specialist doctors, the number of renal units and dialysis centres and the types of treatment, including the drugs, dialysis and psychological support given to patients.

However, there are still many improvements that can be made. One of the most important is to reduce the variation in the treatments that are offered in different parts of the country. All patients, no matter where they live or who their doctor is, should be offered the same level of care and the same choices of treatment. This is not currently the case.

Kidney failure in the UK

The number of people treated for kidney failure in the UK has grown substantially since the late 1990s. The UK Renal Registry (UKRR) was set up by the Renal Association (the specialist kidney doctors' organisation). It acts as a register for all renal units to record information about the patients that they look after so that care across the country can be compared and was started with the intention to improve the care of people in the UK who have kidney failure. It's also very useful for renal units to plan future services, decide what research needs to be done and helps to make new policies to improve services for patients.

At the end of 2016 the Renal Registry reported that there were over 63,000 adult patients receiving renal replacement therapy (RRT) (dialysis or a transplant) in the UK. This has increased from about 15,000 who were known to be receiving treatment in 2000 although at that time only about half of the renal units in the UK reported their activity to the Renal Registry. However, it is safe to say that there are far more patients having dialysis or living with a working kidney transplant than ever before.

The Renal Registry also records what type of treatment people are having. The details of this can be found on their website (https://www.renalreg.org). The records are updated every year.

The registry highlights how different renal units manage their patients. For example, the percentage of patients having Home HD ranges from less than 1% in some places to more than 10% in others. The same is true for PD, where some renal units seem to offer it to more of their patients than do others. The latest report shows a variation of fewer than 4% of dialysis patients having PD in some places and 28% in others.

The same variation is also true for kidney transplants, particularly living donor transplants. The average proportion of people on RRT is nearly 53% of the total. However, some renal units only have about 26% of patients with a transplant. This can be due to many different things, but is mostly due to whether or not the renal unit also has a transplant centre doing the operation itself and therefore looking after more people with a transplant. In fact, the minority of renal units have a transplant centre since the expertise needs to be concentrated to ensure the best outcomes. People with a functioning transplant are then returned to their 'parent' renal unit after a period of time for long-term follow up.

Another factor is the wide variation in the length of time it takes different renal units to place patients on the transplant list; from about 3 months (from the start of dialysis) to over 3 years.

It is worth having a look at the Renal Registry reports on the internet and finding out how well your renal unit is doing, but you should also ask your renal unit team what those numbers mean. These variations may be due to the type of population the renal unit serves, due to organisational factors, but also due to the renal unit's experience, skills and knowledge in looking after people with home-based dialysis or transplants.

Funding

Kidney failure is expensive to treat. Although it affects less than 0.05% of the UK population, about 1.5% of the healthcare budget is spent on treating kidney failure. So kidney failure treatments use proportionately more NHS money than most other diseases. The system is also complex and it is always changing to try and improve it – so by the time you read this it might be different.

In England, renal units are paid for the dialysis treatments or the outpatient visits that they provide through the 'tariff' system. This means that they will get paid for each patient, depending on what treatment they have.

Other aspects of treatment for kidney patients are paid for in different ways. For example, the transport used to get people to and from the dialysis unit for haemodialysis is usually paid for by a local Clinical Commissioning Group (CCG). Other more expensive drugs used for treating anaemia or preventing a transplant from being rejected are paid for by the specialised NHS systems as a top-up to the tariff.

So the money needed to provide the care for someone on haemodialysis comes from several sources. In England, the cost of the dialysis treatment and specialist outpatient visits are paid for by tariff payments direct from NHS England, and they also pay for the EPO. The local CCG pay for any transport to get you to and from hospital, and will also fund any inpatient treatment that you might need. They would also pay for any non-specialist care needed for other reasons. The GP practice will supply and be funded for routine drugs – blood pressure tablets for example – and will carry out any vaccinations. Yes, we said it was complicated!

In the end, it doesn't really matter where the money comes from, as long as patients get the best possible care for the best possible value for money. It's all NHS money funded by the tax payer.

Policy

There have been many different NHS and government documents produced over the years that have attempted to set out what renal services should look like. The first of these was published in January 2004 and was called the Renal National Service Framework (NSF). This policy was initiated by a patient who was then the Chair of the National Kidney Federation (NKF). The NKF led and coordinated the production of this document together with the whole renal community: a wonderful example of how influential patients can be and much of it is still relevant today. It was published in two parts. Part 1 set out five standards which it said the NHS would need to deliver by 2014.

These standards were aimed at helping the health services to manage demand, increase fairness of access – and improve choice and quality in dialysis and kidney transplant services.

Part 2, which was published in 2005, focused on the prevention of ERF, primary care, and end-of-life care.

Ten years after it was published, the NSF expired and a new document was written. Kidney Health – Delivering Excellence built on many of the principles of the NSF and on what had been achieved since its publication. Similar to its predecessor, this document was led by a patient champion, produced with patients, charities and healthcare professionals working together.

This document sets out 16 'ambitions' for how the future of care for people with kidney failure should be organised. The full document can be found on the internet but a summary of the ambitions is below.

1 **Awareness.** To raise the awareness of the risks of kidney disease and what can be done to reduce these risks.

2 **Identification.** To make sure that all people with kidney disease are correctly identified and monitored.

3 **Self-management.** All people with kidney disease are offered as much information as they would like in order to understand and manage their condition.

4 **Person-centred care.** Each person's individual needs, preferences, quality of life, symptom burden and the presence of other medical conditions should all be taken into consideration when planning care.

5 **Acute kidney injury (AKI).** Avoidable harm related to acute kidney injury is prevented in all care settings.

6 **Preparation and choice.** All people approaching end-stage renal disease, or moving from one type of treatment for end-stage renal disease to another, understand and are given sufficient time and support to prepare for a treatment that is suitable for them, chosen from the full range of options.

7 **Equity in transplantation.** Listing for transplantation is based solely on clinical need and suitability, and is not influenced by ethnicity, socio-economic status, or where the potential transplant recipient lives.

8 **Increasing transplantation.** The number of transplants, from both living and deceased donors, is increased so that more patients have the opportunity to receive one.

9 **Living well with a transplant.** A person who receives a transplant is supported to manage their transplant so that they achieve the greatest possible benefit from it.

10 **Dialysis as a specialised service.** Dialysis care (including preparation for dialysis) continues to be commissioned as a specialised service, and is delivered by renal units with the capacity and workforce necessary for all patients to receive high quality dialysis using their chosen method.

11 **Lifestyle on dialysis.** People receive all of the information and education they need to plan and have their dialysis, and are supported to minimise the impact of treatment on their lifestyle and to self-care if they wish.

12 **Care for children and young people.** All children and young people with kidney disease have unrestricted access to a service specifically designed to meet their needs.

13 **Allied services.** All people with kidney disease know about, and have access to, a specialist multi-professional team.

14 **Expert care in rare kidney diseases and in pregnancy.** All people with kidney disease who are contemplating pregnancy have unrestricted access to expert advice and care, wherever they live and whenever it is needed.

15 **Research.** A research strategy for kidney disease is developed, supported by the funding required to design and carry out high quality studies, so that there is a better understanding of the mechanisms of disease and improvements in care quality and outcomes.

16 **Conservative care.** All people who choose not to have dialysis or a transplant are supported by a multi-professional team working closely together to ensure a smooth transition to palliative and end-of life care.

Specialist renal services

Dialysis and kidney transplants have always been treated by the NHS as 'Specialist Services'. This means that the way that services are 'procured' or bought is done by people (commissioners) who have specialist expertise in this area. They also have a responsibility to ensure that the service being delivered by the provider – the renal unit – is safe and effective. Commissioners not only buy the service but they also have a statutory responsibility for the quality of the service. So when they 'hand' money over to the renal unit they will also use information from sources such as the UK Renal Registry to monitor that quality. In turn, the renal unit has a responsibility to collect and report that information. This ensures that both individuals and the system as a whole receive safe and effective care.

Sometimes people get confused by specialised commissioning and specialist care. Commissioning is the process of procuring a service or treatment. It can be defined as specialised or non-specialised. A specialist then oversees a particular problem. So a kidney specialist can look after people with a complicated problem but sometimes it is funded by specialised and sometimes by non-specialised commissioning. If you are reading this book, it is more than likely that you are under a kidney specialist and your kidney treatment is specialised but earlier on, you might have had a kidney specialist but your care was funded by the CCG non-specialised commissioning system. And before that even, you might have had kidney care from your GP or another team – so you would have had non-specialised care funded by non-specialised commissioning. So we don't blame you if you are confused! Perhaps read this paragraph again.

To support the specialised commissioning responsibilities, each specialist area in the NHS in England has a Clinical Reference Group. These groups have been set up to provide clinical advice and leadership to the NHS. The Renal Clinical Reference Group is made up of doctors, commissioners, public health experts, patients and carers. They all use their experiences, knowledge and expertise to advise NHS England on the best ways that the services should be provided.

The Clinical Reference Group produces a 'Service Specification' for each of the areas of therapy. All renal units (in England) should provide the level of care that is set out in these standards. They can be found on the internet on NHS England's website under 'commissioning specialist services'. The CRG is also responsible for setting the commissioning standards, helping the tariff payment system work effectively, dealing with very complex clinical issues that need commissioning solutions and liaising with other parts of the system.

NICE Guidelines and Quality Standards

NICE – the National Institute of Health and Care Excellence – is an organisation that has been set up to help improve health and social care. It does this by looking at all the available evidence for a particular treatment, drug or service and then developing Quality Standards, Clinical or Care Guidelines or Technology Appraisals.

Over the years NICE has produced a number of

relevant guidelines, standards and appraisals which aim to improve care for people with kidney failure. These include a comparison of home and hospital based haemodialysis, standards for PD, renal replacement therapy and treatments following kidney transplants.

You can find out much more detail on the NICE website. All of its publications have a version written specifically for patients and lay people, making them easier to understand.

Getting involved

There are a great many opportunities for patients and relatives or carers to become involved in improving the provision of renal services. In the UK renal care looks very different from where it was a decade ago but there are always things that could be done better. If you want to make suggestions or get involved there are several routes open to you. If NICE guidelines or standards are not being met, or where the dialysis or transplant service specifications are not adhered to, if you think things could be better or something is being missed, patients have a voice. Some suggestions of how you can become involved are:

- Join your local Kidney Patients' Association if there is one. If there is not one, consider whether you might be the person to start one.
- Become a member of the National Kidney Federation which speaks for all kidney patients and has links with the All-Party Parliamentary Group for Kidneys (APPGK) – a group of MPs who fight for resources for kidney patients.
- Another national charity, Kidney Care UK, also provides information and is actively involved in shaping renal services.
- The BKPA has a national network of Advocacy Officers who are available to give practical help, guidance and support to patients and their families. They can help with advice and support for patients who believe they are not being treated fairly.

- Write to your MP or, even better, visit his or her local surgery. Not all politicians are aware of the major problems in British kidney medicine.
- Think about applying to be a member of the Renal Clinical Reference Group.
- Research projects, locally and nationally, are always keen to recruit 'service users' onto project teams. Look at Think Kidneys (www.thinkkidneys.nhs.uk) as an example. Patients are heavily involved in two very important projects working across England – they chair meetings, lead projects and are involved in and run the work at all levels.

KEY FACTS

1 There is evidence of variation between home based and in centre dialysis usage across renal centres in the UK. There is also some evidence that access to transplantation varies between centres.

2 There is more information available, allowing patients to make choices, with regards to their care. It is debatable whether the choices are real.

3 A National Service Framework (NSF) for the care of renal patients was developed in 2005. This work was built on 10 years later when the Kidney Health – Delivering Excellence document was published.

4 Patients have a right to be heard. Joining relevant organisations and writing to the local MP is a good place to start.

GLOSSARY

Words printed in *italic* type have their own glossary entry.

Abdomen The lower part of the trunk, below the chest. Commonly called the tummy or belly.

Access A method of gaining entry to the bloodstream to allow dialysis. Access methods used for *haemodialysis* include a *catheter*, *fistula* or *graft*. Access for *peritoneal dialysis* is a catheter.

Acid A chemical that builds up in the blood in *kidney failure*.

Acute A word meaning short term and of rapid onset, usually requiring a rapid response.

Adequacy This term is used to describe the tests that are used to see how much *dialysis* a patient is getting. Samples of the *dialysis fluid*, blood and samples of *urine* are used to measure the dialysis adequacy.

Albumin A type of *protein* that occurs in the blood. Low blood levels may be linked to malnutrition.

Alfacalcidol A *vitamin D* supplement.

ALG Abbreviation for anti-lymphocyte globulin, a strong treatment against the *rejection* of a *transplant kidney*.

Alkali A substance that is the chemical opposite of an acid.

Alpha blocker A type of *blood pressure* tablet - examples include doxazosin and terazosin.

Amino acids Substances from which *proteins* are built up.

Anaemia A shortage of *red blood cells* in the body, causing tiredness, shortness of breath and pale skin. One of the functions of the *kidneys* is to make *erythropoietin*, which stimulates the *bone marrow* to make *blood cells*. In kidney failure, EPO is not made, and anaemia results.

Angiogram A type of X-ray that uses a special dye to show the *blood vessels*. The dye is put into the blood vessels via a tube that is inserted into the groin and passed up to the *kidneys*.

Angiotensin receptor blocker (ARB) A type of *blood pressure* tablet. Similar to an *ACE inhibitor*.

Angiotensin-converting enzyme (ACE) inhibitor A type of *blood pressure* tablet that can make kidney function worse, although it can be useful in certain situations.

Antibodies Substances that normally help the body to fight infection. They are made by *white blood cells*. After a *transplant*, antibodies can attack the new *kidney* and cause *rejection*.

Antibody incompatible transplantation A technique for increasing the likelihood of successful transplant between a donor and recipient who are not well matched. It involves using particularly strong immunosuppression combined with a dialysis-like process called plasmapharesis and other strong drugs.

Antigen A type of *protein* that occurs on the outer surface of all the cells in a person's body. Antigens act as a 'friendly face' for the cells. The *immune system* normally recognises the friendly face of the body's own *cells*, and does not attack or reject them.

APD Abbreviation for automated *peritoneal dialysis*. A form of peritoneal dialysis that uses a machine to drain the *dialysis fluid* out of the patient and replace it with fresh solution. APD is usually carried out overnight while the patient sleeps.

ARB Short for angiotensin receptor blocker, a type of blood pressure tablet.

Arteries *Blood vessels* that carry blood from the heart to the rest of the body.

Artificial kidney Another name for the *dialyser* or filtering unit of a *dialysis machine*.

ATG Abbreviation for anti-thymocyte globulin, a strong treatment against the *rejection* of a *transplant kidney*.

Atheroma Deposits of *cholesterol* and other fats that cause furring and narrowing of the *arteries* (also called atherosclerosis).

Azathioprine An *immunosuppressant drug* used to prevent the rejection of a *transplant kidney*.

Bacteria A type of germ. Bacteria are microscopically tiny, single-celled organisms capable of independent life. Most are harmless, but some cause disease.

Beta-blockers Tablets that slow down the heart rate and lower blood pressure. Examples are atenolol, bisoprolol and propranolol.

Bicarbonate A substance that is normally present in the blood which is measured in the *biochemistry blood test*. A low blood level of bicarbonate shows there is too much *acid* in the blood.

Biochemistry blood test A test that measures the blood levels of various different substances. Substances measured in people with *kidney failure* usually include *sodium, potassium, glucose, urea, creatinine, bicarbonate, calcium, phosphate* and *albumin*.

Biopsy A test involving the removal of a small piece of an organ or other body *tissue* and its examination under a microscope. A *kidney biopsy* is sometimes used to try and establish the cause of kidney failure. Biopsies are also used to check whether a transplanted *kidney* is being rejected.

Bladder The organ in which *urine* is stored before being passed from the body.

Blood cells The microscopically tiny units that form the solid part of the blood. There are three main types: *red blood cells, white blood cells* and *platelets*.

Blood group An inherited characteristic of *red blood cells*. The common classification is based on whether or not a person has certain *antigens* (called A and B) on their cells. People belong to one of four blood groups, called A, B, AB and O.

Blood level A measurement of the amount of a particular substance in the blood, sometimes expressed in mmol/l (millimoles per litre) or µmol/l (micromoles per litre) of blood.

Blood pressure The pressure the blood exerts against the walls of the arteries as it flows through them. Blood pressure measurements consist of two numbers. The first shows the *systolic blood pressure*, and the second shows the *diastolic blood pressure*. Normal blood pressure is 130/80 or less for most people. One of the functions of the kidney is to help control the blood pressure. In kidney failure, the blood pressure tends to be high.

Cadaveric transplant Another name for a *deceased donor transplant*.

Calcium A mineral that strengthens the bones. It is contained in some foods, including dairy products. It is stored in the bones and is present in the blood. The *kidneys* normally help to keep calcium in the bones. In *kidney failure*, calcium drains out of the bones, and the level of calcium in the blood also falls.

Calcium antagonist A type of blood pressure tablet that can cause 'ankle swelling'. Examples include amlodipine, felodipine and nifedipine.

Calcium carbonate A commonly used type of *phosphate binder*, used to help prevent and treat *renal bone disease*. An example of calcium carbonate is Calcichew. Calcium acetate is sometimes prescribed as an alternative to calcium carbonate.

Candida albicans A fungus that sometimes causes *peritonitis* in patients on *peritoneal dialysis*.

CAPD Abbreviation for continuous ambulatory peritoneal dialysis, a continuous form of *peritoneal dialysis* in which patients perform the exchanges of *dialysis fluid* by hand. The fluid is usually exchanged four times during the day, and is left inside the patient overnight.

Catheter A flexible plastic tube used to enter the interior of the body. A catheter is one of the access options for patients on *haemodialysis*. For patients on *peritoneal dialysis*, a catheter allows *dialysis fluid* to be put into and removed from the *peritoneal cavity*. A catheter may also be used to drain *urine* from the *bladder*.

Cell The cell is the basic structural unit of all living organisms, including humans. It is the smallest unit of life.

Cholesterol A *lipid* (fat) that is a major contributor to *atheroma*.

Chronic A word meaning long term and of slow onset, not usually requiring immediate action.

Chronic kidney disease A long term condition involving a reduction in kidney function. In some people this may be very slight, really no more than natural ageing. However even mild CKD puts people at greater risk of having raised blood pressure and disease in the circulation, even if it does not progress to full scale kidney failure.

Ciclosporin An *immunosuppressant drug* used to prevent the *rejection* of a *transplant kidney*.

CKD A commonly used abbreviation for *chronic kidney disease*.

Clearance The removal of the toxic waste products of food from the body. Clearance is one of the two main functions of the *kidneys*. In *kidney failure*, clearance is inadequate, and *toxins* from food build up in the blood.

CMV Abbreviation for *cytomegalovirus*.

Conservative care programme A planned programme of care for someone who has made a positive decision not to have dialysis or a transplant, to enable them to enjoy the best possible quality of life and to make their own choices during the time they have left to them.

C-reactive protein (CRP) A protein made by the liver and released into the blood within a few hours after tissue injury, the start of an infection or other inflammatory illnesses. It is mostly used to judge if a patient has an infection or not.

Creatinine A waste substance produced by the muscles when they are used. The higher the blood creatinine level, the worse the *kidneys* (or *dialysis* or kidney *transplant*) are working.

Creatinine clearance test A test that measures how effectively the kidneys are working. It involves comparing the creatinine level in the blood to that in the urine. It is normally around 100 mls/min, which approximates to 100 % of normal kidney function. It is similar to the eGFR and is used mainly in the pre-dialysis period.

Cross-match The final blood test before a *transplant operation* is performed. It checks whether the patient has any *antibodies* to the donor *kidney*. The operation can proceed only if the cross-match is negative (i.e. no antibodies are found).

CRP Abbreviation for *C-reactive protein*.

CT scan Abbreviation for a computed tomography scan. An investigation that uses a computer to build up a picture from a series of low-intensity X-rays.

Cytomegalovirus A virus that normally causes only a mild, 'flu-like illness. In people with a *kidney transplant* (and in other people whose immune system is suppressed), CMV can cause a more serious illness affecting the lungs, liver and blood.

Darbepoetin alfa An *erythropoietin stimulating agent* drug.

Deceased donor brain dead A term used to describe a donor whose heart is still beating after *brain death* has occurred. Most, but not all, *deceased donor kidneys* come from brain dead donors.

Deceased donor cardiac dead A donor whose heart is not beating after death, for example if they have had a heart attack in casualty when resuscitation has failed. A few *deceased donor kidneys* come from this source.

Deceased donor kidney A transplant kidney from someone who has died.

Dehydration A condition in which the body does not contain enough water to function properly. Dehydration often occurs with low *blood pressure*, which causes weakness and dizziness.

Diabetes mellitus A condition in which there is too much sugar in the blood. Whether this type of diabetes is controlled by insulin, tablets or diet, it can cause *kidney failure*. This happens most often to people who have had diabetes for longer than 10 years.

Diabetic nephropathy Kidney failure caused by *diabetes mellitus*.

Dialyser The filtering unit of a *dialysis machine*. It provides the *dialysis membrane* for patients on *haemodialysis*. The dialyser removes body wastes and excess water from the blood in a similar way to a normal *kidney*.

Dialysis An artificial process by which the toxic waste products of food and excess water are removed from the body. Dialysis therefore takes over some of the work normally performed by healthy *kidneys*.

Dialysis fluid The liquid that provides the 'container' into which toxic waste products and excess water pass during *dialysis* for removal from the body.

Dialysis machine The machine used to perform *haemodialysis*. It includes a *dialyser*, which filters the patient's blood. The machine helps to pump the patient's blood through the dialyser, and monitors the dialysis process as it takes place.

Dialysis membrane A thin layer of tissue or plastic with many tiny holes in it, through which the process of *dialysis* takes place. In *peritoneal dialysis*, the patient's peritoneum provides the dialysis membrane. For haemodialysis, the dialysis membrane is made of plastic. In each case, the membrane keeps the *dialysis fluid* separate from the blood (essential because dialysis fluid is toxic if it flows directly into the blood). However, the tiny holes in the membrane make it *semi-permeable*, allowing water and various substances to pass through it.

Diastolic blood pressure A *blood pressure* reading taken when the heart is relaxed. It is taken after the *systolic blood pressure* reading and is the second figure in the blood pressure measurement. It should be 80 mmHg or less.

Diffusion A process by which substances pass from a stronger to a weaker solution. Diffusion is one of the key processes in *dialysis* (the other is *ultrafiltration*). During dialysis, body wastes such as *creatinine* pass from the blood into the *dialysis fluid*. At the same time, useful substances such as *bicarbonate* and calcium pass from the dialysis fluid into the blood.

Diuretic drugs The medical name for water tablets. These drugs increase the amount of *urine* that is passed. Two commonly used diuretics are *furosemide* and bumetanide.

Donor A person who donates (gives) an organ to another person (the recipient).

Donor kidney A *kidney* that has been donated.

Doppler scan A type of *ultrasound scan* (sound-wave picture) that provides information about blood flow through the *arteries*.

ECG An abbreviation for *electrocardiogram*.

ECHO An abbreviation for *echocardiogram*.

Echocardiogram (ECHO) A type of ultrasound scan that shows how well the heart is working.

eGFR Estimated *glomerular filtration rate*. The term is generally applied to a test which measures how well the kidneys are working. It is normally around 100 mls/min, which approximates to 100% of normal kidney function. It is similar to the creatinine clearance test and is used mainly in the pre-dialysis period.

Electrocardiogram (ECG) A test that shows the electrical activity within the heart.

End-stage renal failure (ESRF) An alternative name for *established renal failure*.

End-stage renal disease (ESRD) An alternative name for *established renal failure*.

EPO Abbreviation for *erythropoietin*.

ERF Abbreviation for *established renal failure*.

Erythropoietin (EPO) A *hormone*, made by the *kidneys*, which stimulates the *bone marrow* to produce red blood cells.

Erythropoietin stimulating agent (ESA) A type of medication which stimulates the body's own production of *erythropoietin*. ESAs are usually given by injection.

ESA Abbreviation for *erythropoietin stimulating agent*.

Established renal failure (ERF) A term for advanced chronic k*idney failure*. People who develop ERF will die within a few weeks unless treated by *dialysis* or *transplantation*. These treatments control ERF but cannot cure it. Once a patient has developed ERF, they will always have it, even after a *transplant*.

Exit site The point where a *catheter* comes out through the skin. Exit site infections can be a problem for *peritoneal dialysis* patients.

Ferritin A substance in the blood that indicates how much *iron* is present.

Fistula An enlarged *vein*, usually at the wrist or elbow, that gives access to the bloodstream for *haemodialysis*. The fistula is created by a surgeon in a small operation. It is done by joining a vein to an *artery*. This increases the flow of blood through the vein and causes it to enlarge, making it suitable for haemodialysis needles.

Flucloxacillin An antibiotic used to treat exit site infections of *PD* and *haemodialysis catheters*.

Fluid overload A condition in which the body contains too much water. It is caused by drinking too much fluid, or not losing enough. Fluid overload occurs in *kidney failure* because one of the main functions of the *kidneys* is to remove excess water.

Furosemide A commonly-used *diuretic*.

Gentamicin An antibiotic used to treat exit site infections of *PD* and *haemodialysis catheters*.

GFR Abbreviation for glomerular filtration rate. Also the name of a test which indicates how effectively the kidneys get rid of waste by measuring the number of millilitres of blood the kidneys are able to filter in one minute.

Glomerulonephritis Inflammation of the glomeruli, which is one of the causes of *kidney failure*.

Glomerulus One of the tiny filtering units inside the *kidney*.

Glucose A type of sugar. There is normally a small amount of glucose in the blood. This amount is not usually increased in people with *kidney failure* unless they also have *diabetes mellitus*.

Glucose polymer A solution of glucose and other substances, mainly polysaccharides, in which the glucose molecules are very large. Used for oral glucose tolerance tests.

Graft A type of access for *haemodialysis*. The graft is a small plastic tube that connects an *artery* to a *vein*. It is inserted into the arm or leg by a surgeon. *Haemodialysis* needles are inserted into the graft, which can be used many hundreds of times. The term graft is also sometimes used to describe the transplanted kidney.

Haemodiafiltration (HDF) A dialysis method that uses the principles of *diffusion* and convection. This technique allows large amounts water to cross the membrane so that the waste products can be 'flushed' out of the blood.

Haemodialysis A form of *dialysis* in which the blood is cleaned outside the body in a machine called a *dialysis machine*. The machine contains a filter called the dialyser or artificial kidney.

Haemodialysis catheter A plastic tube used to gain access to the bloodstream for *haemodialysis*.

Haemoglobin (Hb) A substance in red blood cells that carries oxygen around the body. Blood levels of haemoglobin are measured to look for *anaemia*. A low Hb level indicates anaemia.

HDF Abbreviation for *haemodiafiltration*.

Hepatitis An infection of the liver, usually caused by a *virus*. Two main types, called hepatitis B and hepatitis C, can be passed on by blood contact. This means that *dialysis* patients, especially those on *haemodialysis*, have an increased risk of getting these infections. Care is taken to reduce this risk, and regular virus checks are made on all kidney patients.

High Dose HD Haemodialysis which is done more often than three times a week for four hours.

HIV Human immunodeficiency virus, the virus that causes AIDS. Tests for HIV are carried out before a patient can have a *transplant*. This is because it may be present and inactive in the patient's body but can be activated by the transplant and *immunosuppressant drugs*.

Home haemodialysis Treatment on a *dialysis* machine installed in a patient's own home.

Hormones Substances that act as chemical messengers in the body. They are produced in parts of the body called endocrine glands. Hormones travel round the body in the blood, and affect how other parts of the body work. For example, parathyroid hormone from the *parathyroid glands* in the neck affects kidney function.

HTA Abbreviation for Human Tissue Authority. This government body must give approval to all *living donor transplants*.

Hypercalcaemia An unusually high level of calcium in the blood. If there is too much calcium in your body, the body will be unable to process it or make use of it, and you may feel very unwell.

Hyperkalaemia An unusually high level of potassium in the blood, which can cause heart problems.

Hyperparathyroidism A disorder in which the parathyroid glands make too much parathyroid hormone.

Hypocalcaemia An unusually low level of calcium in the blood, which can cause problems with the teeth and bones.

Hypokalaemia An unusually low level of potassium in the blood, which can cause weakness, fatigue, muscle cramps and constipation.

Immune system The body's natural defence system. It includes organs (such as the spleen and appendix), lymph nodes (including the 'glands' in the neck) and specialist *white blood cells* called *lymphocytes*. The immune system protects the body from infections, foreign bodies and cancer. To prevent rejection of a *transplant kidney*, patients must take immunosuppressant drugs.

Immunosuppressant drugs A group of drugs used to dampen down the *immune system* to prevent *rejection* of a *transplant kidney*. Commonly used examples are ciclosporin, azathioprine, prednisolone, tacrolimus and mycophenolate mofetil.

Intravenous pyelogram (IVP) A special X-ray of the *kidneys*. A dye that shows up on X-rays is used to show the drainage system of the kidneys. The dye is injected into the patient's arm, travels in the blood to the kidneys, and is passed from the body in the *urine*.

Iron A substance that is necessary to prevent *anaemia*. A low blood *ferritin* indicates low levels of iron in the body.

IVP Abbreviation for *intravenous pyelogram*.

Kidneys The two bean-shaped body organs where *urine* is made. They are located at the back of the body, below the ribs. The two main functions of the kidneys are to remove toxic wastes and to remove excess water from the body.

Kidney biopsy Removal of a small piece of *kidney* through a hollow needle for examination under a microscope. It is needed to diagnose some causes of kidney failure, including nephritis. It is also used to check whether a transplanted kidney is being rejected.

Kidney donor A person who gives a *kidney* for *transplantation*.

Kidney failure A condition in which the *kidneys* are less able than normal to perform their functions of removing toxic wastes, removing excess water, helping to control *blood pressure*, helping to control *red blood cell* manufacture and helping to keep the bones strong and healthy. Kidney failure can be *acute* or *chronic*. Advanced chronic kidney failure is called *established renal failure or ERF*.

Kidney machine Another name for a *dialysis machine*.

Kidney transplant An alternative name for a *transplant kidney*, or for the *transplant operation* during which a new kidney is given to the recipient.

LFTs Abbreviation for *liver function tests*.

Line infection A name for an infection of a *haemodialysis catheter* (or line).

Lipids Another name for fats. People with *kidney failure* tend to have raised lipid levels in the blood.

Liver function tests (LFTs) Blood tests that show how well the liver is working. They often appear at the bottom of the *biochemistry blood test* results. Some people with *kidney failure* also have liver problems.

Living donor transplant A *transplant kidney* removed from someone who is alive.

Living related transplant (LRT) A *transplant kidney* donated (given) by a living relative of the recipient. A well-matched living related transplant is likely to last longer than either a *living unrelated transplant* or a *deceased donor transplant*.

Living unrelated transplant (LURT) A *kidney transplant* from a living person who is biologically unrelated to the recipient (such as a husband or wife).

Lymphocytes Specialist *white blood cells* that form part of the *immune system*.

Malnutrition Loss of body weight, usually due to not eating enough (especially foods containing protein and energy). Malnutrition is the major nutritional problem of dialysis patients.

Marker A substance that is known to occur in the presence of another substance. Both creatinine and urea are markers for many less easily measurable substances in the blood. The higher the blood levels of these marker substances, the higher also are the levels of harmful toxins in the blood.

Membrane A thin, skin-like layer, resembling a piece of 'cling film'. The *peritoneum* is a natural membrane used as the *dialysis membrane* in *peritoneal dialysis*. In *haemodialysis*, the dialysis membrane is a plastic membrane inside the *dialyser*.

mmol/l Abbreviation for millimoles per litre. A unit used to measure the blood levels of many substances. *Creatinine* is measured in smaller units called micromoles per litre (μmol/l).

Molecule The smallest unit that a substance can be divided into without causing a change in the chemical nature of the substance.

MRI scan Abbreviation for magnetic resonance imaging scan, a scanning technique that uses magnetism, radiowaves and a computer to produce high-quality pictures of the body's interior.

mycophenolate mofetil An *immunosuppressant drug*, sometimes used as an alternative to *azathioprine*.

Nephr- Prefix meaning relating to the *kidneys*.

Nephrectomy An operation to remove a kidney from the body. A bilateral nephrectomy is an operation to remove both kidneys.

Nephritis A general term for inflammation of the *kidneys*. Also used as an abbreviation for *glomerulonephritis*. A *kidney biopsy* is needed to diagnose nephritis.

Nephrologist Another name for a kidney doctor.

Nephrology The study of the *kidneys*.

NHS Blood and Transplant NHS BT coordinates the provision of organs for transplants in the UK. They are responsible for the retrieval and matching of organs via the NHS Organ Donor Register and National Transplant Register.

NICE Abbreviation for National Institute for Health and Care Excellence, and the name by which this body is commonly known. NICE looks at whether new treatments are effective and issues guidelines for good practice.

Nuclear medicine scan Another name for a *radio-isotope scan*. Examples include DMSA, DTPA, and MAG-3 scans.

Obstructive nephropathy Blockage to the drainage system of the *kidney*, through which the *urine* passes.

Oedema An abnormal build-up of fluid, mainly water, in the body. People with *kidney failure* are prone to *fluid overload*, leading to oedema.

OKT3 Abbreviation for orthoclone K T-cell receptor antibody, a strong treatment for the rejection of a transplant.

Organ A part of the body that consists of different types of *tissue*, and that performs a particular function. Examples include the *kidneys*, heart and brain.

Osmosis The process by which water moves from a weaker to a stronger solution through tiny holes in a *semi-permeable* membrane. In *peritoneal dialysis*, it is osmosis that causes excess water to pass from the blood into the *dialysis fluid*.

Paired and pooled donation Two or more living donor transplants made possible by unmatched donor-recipient pairs getting together to ensure that each recipient ends up with a kidney with which they are better matched.

Parathormone (PTH) Another name for parathyroid hormone.

Parathyroidectomy An operation to remove the *parathyroid glands*.

Parathyroid glands Four pea-sized glands near the thyroid gland at the front of the neck.

Parathyroid hormone (PTH) A hormone produced by the *parathyroid glands*, which helps control blood levels of *calcium*. When the level of calcium in the blood is low, PTH boosts it by causing calcium to drain from the bones into the blood. PTH is the best long-term indicator of the severity of *renal bone disease*.

PCKD Abbreviation for p*olycystic kidney disease*.

PD Abbreviation for *peritoneal dialysis*.

PD catheter A plastic tube through which *dialysis fluid* for *peritoneal dialysis* is put into, and removed from, the *peritoneal cavity*. The catheter is about 30 centimetres (12 inches) long, and as wide as a pencil. A small operation is needed to insert the catheter permanently into the *abdomen*.

Peritoneal cavity The area between the two layers of the *peritoneum* inside the *abdomen*. The peritoneal cavity contains the abdominal organs, including the stomach, liver and bowels. It normally contains only about 100 ml of liquid, but expands easily to provide a reservoir for the *dialysis fluid* in *peritoneal dialysis*.

Peritoneal dialysis (PD) A form of dialysis that takes place inside the patient's *peritoneal cavity*, using the *peritoneum* as the *dialysis membrane*. Bags of *dialysis fluid*, containing *glucose* (sugar) and various other substances, are drained in and out of the peritoneal cavity via a PD catheter.

Peritoneal equilibration test (PET) A measurement of the rate at which *toxins* pass out of the blood into the dialysis fluid during *peritoneal dialysis* (PD). Patients are described as 'high transporters' if the toxins move quickly and 'low transporters' if the toxins move more slowly. The test is used to assess a patient's suitability for different types of PD.

Peritoneum A natural membrane that lines the inside of the wall of the *abdomen* and that covers all the abdominal organs (the stomach, bowels, liver, etc.). The peritoneum provides the *dialysis membrane* for *peritoneal dialysis*. It has a large surface area, contains many tiny holes and has a good blood supply.

Peritonitis Inflammation of the *peritoneum*, caused by an infection. People on *peritoneal dialysis* risk getting peritonitis if they touch the connection between their peritoneal dialysis catheter and the bags of *dialysis fluid*. Most attacks are easily treated with antibiotic drugs.

PET In this context, an abbreviation for *peritoneal equilibrium test*. (The abbreviation PET in PET scan can also be short for positron emission tomography.)

Phosphate A mineral that helps *calcium* to strengthen the bones. Phosphate is obtained from foods such as dairy products, nuts and meat. The *kidneys* normally help to keep the right amount of phosphate in the blood. In *kidney failure*, phosphate tends to build up in the blood. High phosphate levels occur with low calcium levels in people with *renal bone disease*.

Phosphate binders Tablets that help prevent a build-up of *phosphate* in the body. Phosphate binders combine with phosphate in food so that it passes it out of the body in the faeces.

PKD Abbreviation for polycystic kidney disease

Polycystic kidney disease A disease that runs in families, in which both kidneys are full of cysts (abnormal fluid-filled lumps). It is one of the causes of *kidney failure.*

Potassium A mineral that is normally present in the blood, and which is measured in the *biochemistry blood test.* Too much or too little potassium can be dangerous, causing the heart to stop. People with *kidney failure* may need to restrict the amount of potassium in their diet.

Prednisolone A steroid used to prevent or treat the rejection of a *transplant kidney.*

Proteins Chemical components of the body, formed from *amino acids.* The body needs supplies of protein in the diet to build muscles and to repair itself.

PTH Abbreviation for *parathyroid hormone.*

Pulmonary oedema A serious condition in which fluid builds up in the lungs, causing breathlessness. People with *kidney failure* develop pulmonary oedema if *fluid overload* is not treated promptly.

Pyelonephritis Inflammation of the drainage system of the *kidneys,* one of the causes of *kidney failure.* It can be diagnosed by an ultrasound scan, an *intravenous pyelogram* or a *nuclear medicine scan.*

Radio-isotope scan A method of obtaining pictures of the body's interior, also called a radio-nuclide scan or *nuclear medicine scan.* A small amount of a mildly radioactive substance is either swallowed or injected into the bloodstream. The substance gathers in certain parts of the body, which then show up on pictures taken by a special machine.

Recipient In the context of *transplantation,* a person who receives an organ from another person (the *donor*).

Red blood cells Cells in the blood which carry oxygen from the lungs around the body.

Reflux nephropathy A condition in which *urine* passes back up from the *bladder,* through the *ureters,* to the *kidneys,* where it can cause infections. It occurs because a valve that normally prevents the backflow of urine from the bladder is faulty. Reflux nephropathy is one of the causes of *kidney failure.*

Rejection The process by which a patient's *immune system* recognises a *transplant kidney* (or other transplanted organ) as not its 'own', and then tries to destroy it and remove it from the body. Rejection can be *acute* or *chronic.*

Renal bone disease A complication of *kidney failure,* in which bone health is affected by abnormally low blood levels of *calcium* and *vitamin D,* and high levels of phosphate. Without treatment, renal bone disease can result in bone pain and fractures.

Renal unit A hospital department that treats disorders of the *kidneys.*

Renovascular disease Atheroma affecting the b*lood vessels* that supply the kidneys. Renovascular disease is a common cause of *kidney failure* in older patients.

Residual renal function (RRF) The amount of kidney function that a patient on dialysis has. This varies from patient to patient. It is likely the RRF will reduce over a period of time, and in many patients, it eventually disappears altogether. A *creatinine clearance test* is used to assess RRF.

Rifampicin An *antibiotic drug,* commonly used to treat long-term *exit site* infections of *peritoneal dialysis* catheters.

Rigors Cold shivers that sometimes occur with a fever. They can be a symptom of an infected *haemodialysis catheter*.

RRF Abbreviation for *residual renal function*.

Satellite haemodialysis unit A place where some patients go for *haemodialysis* away from the main hospital *renal unit*. Satellite units have relatively few nurses and are suitable only for healthy patients who do some of the haemodialysis preparation themselves. These units tend to be more readily accessible to patients than most main hospital buildings.

Scan One of several techniques for obtaining pictures of the body's interior without using conventional X-rays. Examples include *CT scans, MRI scans, radio-isotope scans* and *ultrasound scans*.

Semi-permeable An adjective, often used to describe a *membrane*, meaning that it will allow some but not all substances to pass through it. Substances with smaller *molecules* will pass through the holes in the membrane, whereas substances with larger molecules will not.

Shared care A process of supporting you in undertaking elements of your own care - e.g. monitoring your own blood pressure, preparing a machine, inserting your own disalysis needles, carrying out your PD fluid exchanges.

Sirolimus An immunosuppressant drug that is used as an alternative to *ciclosporin* or *tacrolimus*.

Sodium A mineral that is normally present in the blood, and which is measured in the *biochemistry blood test*. Sodium levels are not usually a problem for people with *kidney failure* and are quite easily controlled by *dialysis*.

Sphygmomanometer The instrument used to measure *blood pressure*.

Staphylococcus One of a group of bacteria responsible for various infections (often called 'staph' infections). A common cause of *peritonitis* in patients on *peritoneal dialysis*, and of *line infections* in *haemodialysis* patients.

Statins A group of drugs that reduce lipid levels in the blood, especially cholesterol. Examples include atorvastatin and simvastatin.

Systolic blood pressure A blood pressure reading taken when the heart squeezes as it beats. The systolic blood pressure is measured before the *diastolic blood pressure* reading and is the first figure in a blood pressure measurement.

Tacrolimus An *immunosuppressant drug*, also known as FK506, which is an alternative to *ciclosporin* or *sirolimus*.

Tissue A collection of similar cells that share a similar function, such as skin cells or *kidney* cells.

Tissue type A set of inherited characteristics on the surface of cells. Each person's tissue type has six components (three from each parent). Although there are only three main sorts of tissue type characteristic (called A, B and DR), each of these comes in 20 or more different versions. Given the large number of possibilities, it is unusual for there to be an exact tissue type match between a *transplant kidney* and its recipient. However, the more characteristics that match, the more likely a *transplant* is to succeed.

Tissue typing A blood test that identifies a person's *tissue type*.

Toxins Poisons. One of the main functions of the *kidneys* is to remove toxins from the blood (a process known as *clearance*).

Transplant A term used to mean either a transplant kidney (or other transplant organ) or a *transplant operation*.

Transplantation The replacement of an organ in the body by another person's organ. Many organs can now be successfully transplanted, including the kidneys, liver, bowel, heart, lungs, pancreas, skin and bones.

Transplant kidney A *kidney* removed from one person (the donor) and given to another person (the recipient). Transplant kidneys may be either *deceased donor transplants* or *living donor transplants*.

Transplant operation The surgical operation by which a patient is given a donated organ. The operation to insert a *transplant kidney* takes about 2–3 hours. The new *kidney* is placed lower in the *abdomen* than the patient's own kidneys, which are usually left in place. Blood vessels attached to the transplant kidney are connected to the patient's blood supply, and the new kidney's *ureter* is connected to the patient's bladder.

Transplant waiting list A system that seeks to find the 'right' transplant organ for the 'right' patient. It is co-ordinated nationally by *NHS Blood and Transplant*, whose computer compares patients' details (including *blood group and tissue type*) with those of deceased donor organs that become available. The average waiting time for a *cadaveric transplant kidney* is about three years.

Tunnel infection A possible problem for patients on *peritoneal dialysis* (PD). It occurs when an infection spreads from the *exit site* into the 'tunnel' (i.e. the route of the PD catheter through the abdominal wall).

Ultrafiltration The removal of excess water from the body. Ultrafiltration is one of the two main functions of the *kidneys*. In *kidney failure*, problems with ultrafiltration result in *fluid overload*. *Dialysis* provides an alternative means of ultrafiltration.

Ultrasound scan A method of obtaining pictures of internal organs, such as the *kidneys*, or of an unborn baby, using sound waves. A device that sends out sound waves is held against the body. The sound waves produce echoes, which the scanner detects and builds up into pictures.

Under-dialysis Not having enough *dialysis*. If a dialysis patient does not achieve target blood levels for *creatinine*, the symptoms of *kidney failure* are likely to return. The amount of dialysis will then have to be increased.

Urea A substance made by the liver. It is one of the waste products from food that builds up in the blood when someone has kidney failure. Like *creatinine*, urea is a marker for other more harmful substances. The higher the urea level, the worse is the kidney failure.

Ureters The tubes that take urine from the *kidneys* to the *bladder*.

Urethra The body's tube that takes *urine* from the *bladder* to the outside of the body.

Urinary catheter A plastic tube inserted into the *bladder* for the removal of *urine*.

Urine The liquid produced by the *kidneys*, consisting of the toxic waste products of food and the excess water from the blood.

Vancomycin An antibiotic drug, commonly used to treat *peritonitis*, long-term *exit site* infections (of *peritoneal dialysis* catheters) and line (*haemodialysis* catheter) infections.

Vasodilator drugs Tablets that lower the *blood pressure* by making the blood vessels wider, so that the blood can flow through them more easily.

Veins *Blood vessels* which carry blood from the body back to the heart.

Virus A type of germ responsible for a range of mild and serious illnesses. Viruses are much smaller than *bacteria* and usually reproduce inside the cells of other living organisms.

Vitamin D A chemical that helps the body to absorb calcium from the diet. Blood levels of vitamin D are usually low in people with *kidney failure*.

Water tablets The common name for *diuretic drugs*.

White blood cells *Cells* in the blood that normally help to fight infection. They are part of the *immune system*. After a *kidney* transplant, they can be a 'bad thing', as they may attack (reject) the new kidney.

Xenotransplantation The transplanting of tissues or organs from one animal into a human or other type of animal.

FURTHER READING

You will find many information leaflets from Kidney Care UK and the National Kidney Federation. A DVD featuring patients and kidney specialists and entitled Living with Kidney Disease is available from Kidney Research UK or the NKF. The following books are also likely to be helpful:

Dialysing for Life. Jacob van Noordwijk. Kluwer Academic Publishers.

Eating Well for Kidney Health. Helena Jackson, Claire Green and Gavin James. Class Health.

Eating Well With Kidney Failure. Helena Jackson, Annie Cassidy and Gavin James. Class Health.

High Blood Pressure: Answers at your fingertips. Professor Tom Fahey, Professor Deirdre Murphy and Dr Julian Tudor Hart. Class Health.

Kidney Failure: the facts. Dr Stewart A Cameron. Oxford University Press.

Kidney Matters, the magazine of Kidney Care UK, published quarterly. Available for free (see website for details).

Kidney Transplants Explained. Dr Andy Stein, Dr Rob Higgins and Janet Wild. Class Health.

Living Well with Kidney Failure. Juliet Auer. Class Health.

Oxford Handbook of Dialysis. Jeremy Levy, Julie Morgan and Edwina Brown. Oxford University Press.

Renal Registry Report 2015. Available from the Renal Registry website at https://www.renalreg.org/reports/2015-eighteenth-annual-report (Previous years' reports are available from the same site.)

Type 1 Diabetes: Answers at your fingertips. Dr Charles Fox and Dr Anne Kilvert. Class Health.

Type 2 Diabetes: Answers at your fingertips. Dr Charles Fox and Dr Anne Kilvert. Class Health.

Whose Kidney is it Now? And other questions asked by potential live donors. Sue Rabbitt Roff. Downloadable as a PDF from the NKF website: www.kidney.org.uk

USEFUL ADDRESSES AND WEBSITES

Addresses are correct at time of going to press, but please note that all are subject to change from time to time.

Action on Smoking and Health (ASH)
6th Floor, Suites 59-63
New House
67-68 Hatton Garden
London EC1N 8JY
Tel: 020 7404 0242
Website: www.ash.org.uk
Information on how smoking affects medical conditions.

Age UK
Tavis House
1-6 Tavistock Square
London WC1H 9NA
Tel: 0800 055 6112
Website: www.ageuk.org.uk
A new organisation combining Age Concern and Help the Aged. The Age UK family also includes Age Cymru, Age NI and Age Scotland. Provides advice and publications on a range of subjects for older people.

British Association of Counselling and Psychotherapy
BACP
15 St John's Business Park
Lutterworth
Leicestershire LE17 4HB
Tel: 01455 883300
Website: www.bacp.co.uk
Send s.a.e. for information about counselling services in your area, and publications list.

British Heart Foundation
Lyndon Place
2096 Coventry Road
Sheldon
Birmingham B26 3YU
Tel: 0300 330 3322
Website: www.bhf.org.uk
Funds research, promotes education and raises money for equipment to treat people with heart disease.

Carers UK
20 Great Dover Street
London SE1 4LX
Tel: 020 7378 4999
Advice line: 0808 808 7777
Website: www.carersuk.org
Offers information and support to all people who have to care for others due to medical or other problems.

Citizens Advice
Website: www.citizensadvice.org.uk
National charity offering a wide variety of practical, legal and financial advice through its network of local branches throughout the UK and its Adviceguide website.

Carers Trust
32-36 Loman Street
London SE1 0EH
Tel: 0300 772 9600
Website: www.carers.org
Supports and delivers high quality services (including respite care) for carers and people in need via its local branches.

CRUSE Bereavement Care
PO Box 800
Richmond
Surrey TW9 1RG
Tel: 0208 939 9530
Helpline: 0808 808 1677
Website: www.cruse.org.uk
Offers information and practical advice. Sells literature and has local branches that provide one-to-one counselling to people who have been bereaved. Runs training in bereavement counselling for professionals.

Department of Health and Social Care
39 Victoria Street
London
SW1H 0EU
Website: www.dh.gov.uk

Diabetes UK
Wells Lawrence House
126 Back Church Lane
London E1 1FH
Tel: 0345 123 2399
Fax: 020 7424 1001
Website: www.diabetes.org.uk
Provides advice and information for people with diabetes and their families; has local support groups.

Disability Rights UK
Plexal
14 East Bay Lane
Here East
Queen Elizabeth Olympic Park
Stratford
London E20 3BS
Tel: 0330 995 0400
Campaigns to improve the rights and care of people with a disability. Sells special key to access locked public toilets for the disabled.

DVLA (Drivers and Vehicles Licensing Authority)
Drivers Medical Enquiries
Swansea SA99 1TU
Tel: 0300 790 6806
Website: www.dvla.gov.uk
Government office providing advice for drivers with special needs.

Globaldialysis
Website: www.globaldialysis.com
Gives details of holidays and travel information for dialysis patients.

Human Tissue Authority
Website: www.hta.gov.uk
This organisation was set up to regulate the removal, storage, use and disposal of human bodies, organs and tissue from both living and deceased donors.

Jobcentre Plus
Website: www.los.direct.gov.uk
The section of the Department for Work and Pensions that supports people looking for work and distributes some welfare benefits, including Jobseeker's Allowance and Employment and Support Allowance. Local Jobcentre Plus offices can be found in your local telephone directory or on the Jobcentre Plus website.

Kidney Cancer UK
The Old Coach House
High Street
Harston
Cambridge
CB22 7PZ
Tel: 01223 870008
Website: www.kcuk.org.uk
Information and support for people with kidney cancer and their carers. Chat room available via the website.

Kidney Care UK
3 The Windmills
St Mary's Close
Turk Street
Alton GU34 1EF
Tel: 01420 541424
Website: www.kidneycareuk.org
Provides information and advice to people with kidney illnesses throughout the UK. Grants available.

Kidney Patient Information Website
Website: www.kidneypatientguide.
org.uk
*Information for patients with kidney
failure, and those who care for them.*

Kidney Research UK
Nene Hall
Lynch Wood Park
Peterborough PE2 6FZ
Helpline: 0300 3031100
Website: www.kidneyresearchuk.org
*Funds research into kidney disease, its
causes and treatment. Works to raise
awareness of kidney disease.*

Macmillan Cancer Support
89 Albert Embankment
London SE1 7UQ
Tel: 020 7840 7840
Fax: 020 7840 7841
Helpline: 0808 808 0000
Website: www.macmillan.org.uk
*Helps cancer patients, families and
carers with practical and emotional
support.*

Medic-Alert Foundation
Medic-Alert House
327–329 Upper Fourth Street
Milton Keynes
MK9 1EH
E-mail: info@medicalert.org.uk
*Offers a selection of jewellery with
internationally recognised medical
symbol: 24 hour emergency phoneline.*

**MIND (National Association for
Mental Health)**
15–19 Broadway
Stratford
London E15 4BQ
Tel: 020 8519 2122
Helpline: 0300 123 3393
Website: www.mind.org.uk
*Mental health organisation
working for a better life for everyone
experiencing mental distress. Has
information and offers support via
local branches.*

National Kidney Federation
The Point
Coach Road
Shireoaks
Worksop
Notts S81 8BW
Tel: (01909) 544999
Fax: (01909) 481723
Helpline: 0800 169 09 36
Website: www.kidney.org.uk
*Aims to promote, throughout the
United Kingdom, the welfare of people
suffering from kidney disease or renal
failure, and those relatives and friends
who care for them.*

NHS 24
Scotland's national Telehealth and
Telecare organisation
Tel: 111 (free)

NHS Blood and Transplant
NHSBT
Oak House
Reeds Crescent
Watford
Hertfordshire WD24 4QN
Tel: 0300 123 2323
Website: www.nhsbt.uk
*Provides information about donating
organs and how patients can benefit
from organ donation.*

**National Institute for Health and
Care Excellence (NICE)**
Website: www.nice.org.uk
*The organisation responsible for
providing national guidance on drugs
and treatments offered in the NHS.*

Outsiders
West End
Redwood Farm
Barrow Gurney
Avon BS48 3RE
Tel: 07770 884 985
Website: www.outsiders.org.uk
*A national self-help organisation
that provides advice about sexual
relationships to people with
disabilities.*

Patients Association
PO Box 935
Harrow
Middlesex HA1 3YJ
Tel: 020 8423 9111
Helpline: 020 8433 8999
Website: www.patients-association.
org.uk
Provides advice on patients' rights.

Patient View
Website: www.patientview.org
Ask your renal unit about access to this site, which will enable you to view your own results and care pathways on the Internet.

PKD Charity
91 Royal College
London NW1 0SE
Tel: 020 7387 0543
Helpline: 0300 111 1234
Website: www.pkdcharity.org.uk
Supports people affected by APKD, their families and carers. Raises awareness and funds research.

Registered Nursing Homes Association
Derek Whittaker House
Tunnel Lane
Off Lifford Lane
Kings Norton
Birmingham B30 3JN
Tel: 0121 451 1088
Freephone: 0800 0740 194
Website: www.rnha.co.uk
Information about registered nursing homes in your area that meet the standards set by the Association.

Relate
Premier House
Carolina Court
Lakeside
Doncaster DN4 5RA
Tel: 0300 100 1234
(or see your phonebook for local branch)
Website: www.relate.org.uk
Offers relationship counselling via local branches, and publishes information on health, sexual, self-esteem, depression, bereavement and remarriage issues.

Sharing Haemodialysis Care
Website: www.shareddialysis-care.org.uk
Information and resources about the Shared HD care project.

Think Kidneys
Website: www.thinkkidneys.nhs.uk
National programmes led by the renal community and the UK Renal Registry.

UK Renal Registry
Southmead Hospital
Bristol BS10 5NB
Tel: 0117 414 8150
Website: www.renalreg.com
Collects, analyses and presents data about the incidence, clinical management and outcome of renal disease.

Vitalise
212 Business Design Centre
52 Upper Street
London N1 0QH
Tel: 0303 303 0145
Website: www.revitalise.org.uk
Formerly known as the Winged Fellowship Trust, provides holidays and respite care for disabled people and their carers.

INDEX

Priority order form

Cut out or photocopy this form and send it to:

Class Publishing Priority Service, The Exchange, Express Park, Bristol Road, Bridgwater, TA6 4RR
Tel: 01278 427800 or email post@class.co.uk

Please send me urgently
(tick below)

Post included price per copy (UK only)

❏ **Kidney Failure Explained** £28.49
(ISBN: 978 1 85959 792 7)

❏ **Eating Well for Kidney Health** £23.49
(ISBN: 978 1 85959 204 5)

❏ **Eating Well with Kidney Failure** £23.49
(ISBN: 978 1 85959 116 1)

❏ **Living Well with Kidney Failure** £21.49
(ISBN: 978 185959 112 3)

❏ **Kidney Dialysis and Transplants: Answers at your fingertips** £21.49
(ISBN: 978 185959 046 1)

❏ **Kidney Transplants Explained** £23.49
(ISBN: 978 1 85959 193 2)

❏ **Type 1 Diabetes: Answers at your fingertips** £21.49
(ISBN: 978 185959 175 8)

❏ **Type 2 Diabetes: Answers at your fingertips** £21.49
(ISBN: 978 185959 323 3)

TOTAL _____

Easy ways to pay

Cheque: I enclose a cheque payable to Class Publishing for £

Credit card: please debit my ❏ Mastercard ❏ Visa ❏ Amex

Number _____ Expiry date _____ CSV- 3 digits _____

Name _____

My address for delivery is _____

Town _____ County _____ Postcode _____

Telephone number (in case of query) _____

Credit card billing address if different from above _____

_____

If you have any feedback on Class Health publications please email: post@class.co.uk